THE **FOOD DOCTOR** DIET

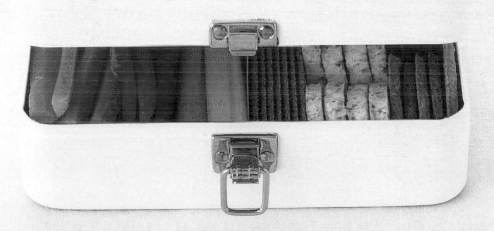

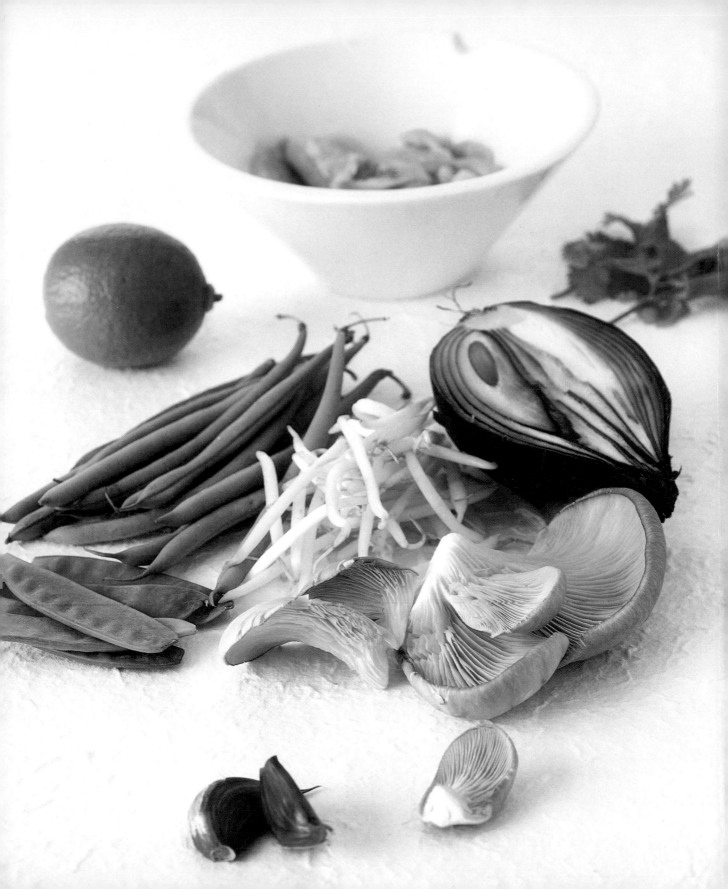

THE FOOD DOCTOR DIET

Ian Marber, MBANT, Dip ION

For more information
from The Food Doctor visit
www.thefooddoctor.com

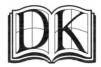

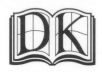

London, New York, Melbourne,
Munich, Delhi

For my father,
with love and heartfelt admiration

Project editor	Susannah Steel
Designer	Mark Cavanagh
Managing editor	Stephanie Farrow
DTP designer	Sonia Charbonnier
Production controller	Stuart Masheter
Art director	Carole Ash
Category publisher	Mary-Clare Jerram
Food stylist and	
home economist	Pippin Britz
Photographer	Sian Irvine

Note to readers:
Do not attempt the Seven-day Diet if you
are pregnant, or 16 years old or under.
Please consult your doctor first if you have
a diagnosed medical condition.

First published in Great Britain in 2003
by Dorling Kindersley Limited,
80 Strand, London WC2R 0RL
A Penguin Group
6 8 10 9 7 5

A CIP catalogue record for this
book is available from The British Library
ISBN 1 4053 0142 2
Colour reproduction by Colourscan, Singapore
Printed and bound in Portugal by Printer Portuguesa

Discover more at
www.dk.com

Contents

Seven-day diet

Plan for life

The ten principles

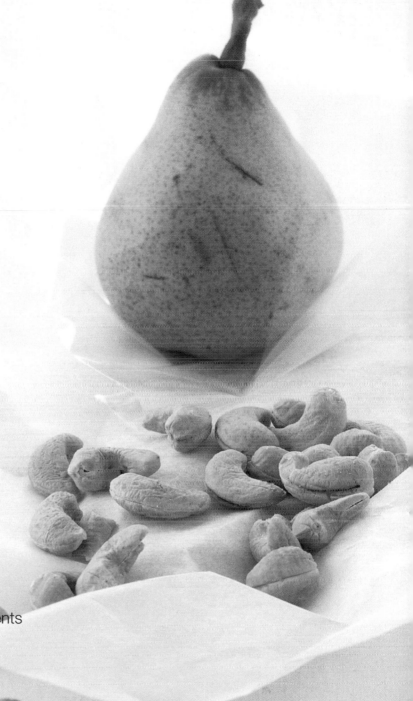

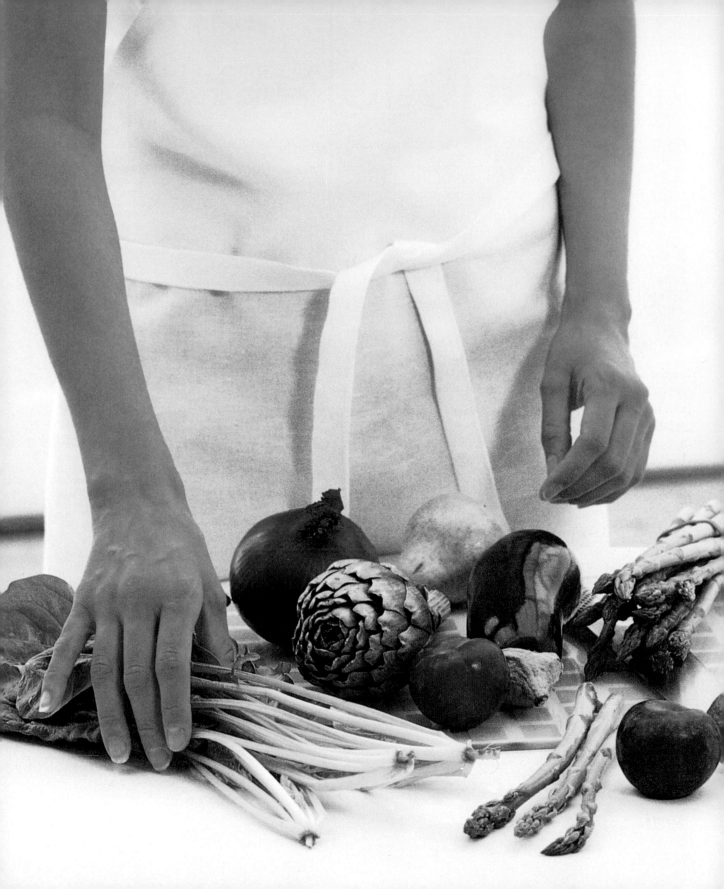

Introduction

My career as a nutrition consultant has encompassed everything from giving individual consultations and workshops to writing newspaper columns and magazine articles and appearing on television and radio. And yet I know that the first question people will always ask me is, "How do I lose weight?"

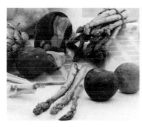

Before you think that I have inherited a gene that helps me to stay trim, and that I don't know how it feels to be frustrated and uncomfortable about weight issues, you should know that I have battled with my own weight over the years. There have been times when I have felt under immense pressure to diet since, given my profession, I am supposed to be slim. It has taken me some time to work out how to maintain a comfortable weight, and I am sure that I could lose a few more pounds. Nevertheless, I have come to terms with the fact that the weight I want to be, or feel I should be, isn't always a realistic aim.

The dieting cycle

I have been asked to write diet books before, but I shied away because I didn't want to jump on any bandwagons. However, having worked with so many clients who have followed faddy diets, "quick fixes" and potentially unsafe weight-loss programmes, I feel that now is the right time to debunk the myths and help people achieve their goals.

Let me start with some semantics. Our understanding of the word "diet" is as a short-term eating programme with a beginning, a middle and an end. You follow the regime, lose weight, then revert to your old eating habits and so gain weight. You blame the diet – "It didn't work for me" – buy another book or join another club, and off you go again. You gain the weight back – and maybe more – in the interim, of course, and then turn to another diet, hoping that this one will work for you. There is one winner and one loser in this cycle: you lose money and self-esteem, while the diet industry gains another long-term customer.

I have read nearly every diet book there is, and while many diets have some really good elements to them, they can be pretty hard to understand without a degree in biochemistry, and are difficult to follow unless you don't mind endlessly weighing food. But that's not the worst of it. Some diet experts suggest eating particular foods, or insist that their programme will fail unless you eat obscure foods that you have never heard of, and that you can't find in your local market. It's no wonder that so many people fail to lose weight.

What's different about this diet?

The Food Doctor weight loss plan focuses primarily on achieving good health, especially that of the digestive system. I believe that if you follow my plan, and also make good digestive health your main aim, you should succeed in your goal to lose weight and feel great.

I also believe that by understanding just how good health can be achieved, you will be able to apply the plan to your own lifestyle, taking into account your income, working hours, commitments and social life.

If you follow my plan, and also make **good digestive health** your **main aim,** you should **succeed** in your goal to **lose weight** and feel **great**

Digestion – a quick tour

I believe that a healthy digestive system enhances the absorption of nutrients, and can go a long way towards reducing cravings for sugary, processed foods and drinks. So let me first explain briefly about the process of digestion. By the way, turn to the glossary *(see pp.138–39)* if you are unsure of any terms or words.

Digestion is the process of breaking down food for the body to absorb. As we eat, the combination of enzymes in our saliva and the process of chewing start to break down the bonds that hold food together. However, saliva

I believe that digestive problems occur if the efficient workings of the digestive system are impaired by the sort of diet and lifestyle that have probably been largely responsible for excess weight in the first place. A diet that is high in refined sugars and saturated fats, combined with lack of chewing and high stress levels, can create an internal environment in which foods are not broken down properly and nutrients are poorly absorbed. Our energy levels can also soar and dip sharply in response to a high intake of refined sugars, which can lead to sugar cravings that we interpret as hunger – and so the cycle continues.

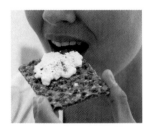

Lesson number one is to **chew** your food **properly** in order that your body can **digest** it **effectively**

is relatively mild and is limited in its effectiveness, so you must chew well. If you don't chew your food, you are at a disadvantage, the consequences of which are explained in more detail below. If you do chew each mouthful properly, your body can begin to digest it more effectively.

Once you have swallowed your food, it passes on down to the stomach (which is located under the rib cage and not at the navel, as most people think). Here it is churned many times with a variety of substances, most notably with hydrochloric acid, which is a potent acid that further breaks down the bonds that hold food together. Yet however strong hydrochloric acid is, if you haven't chewed your food properly, it probably won't be broken down as well as it could while in the stomach.

At the end of this stage the partly-digested food is known as chyme, an acid pulp that is released through a valve into the intestines. It is in the intestines that the nutrients are filtered out and absorbed into the bloodstream: the chyme is constantly turned over and passed back and forth in each area of intestine so that it is exposed to tiny little intestinal protrusions called villi, which filter out the nutrients. The chyme continues along the intestines as if on a conveyor belt until all the nutrients have been taken out and only waste is left, which is then released from the body as faeces.

Friends and foes

Lurking inside the intestines are countless bacteria that also have a profound effect on your digestive health. Some bacteria, called *Lactobacillus acidophilus* and *Lactobacillus bifidum bacterium*, are beneficial to the intestines, some are innocuous and others, in large amounts, can be defined as potentially unfriendly bacteria, such as the *Citrobacter freundii, Klebsiella pneumoniae* and *Bacillus* species. So the right balance of bacteria is crucial to your digestive health. A stool analysis arranged by your doctor or nutrition consultant will reveal just how well your digestive system is working.

Checking your internal health

You can get a clue to your internal health just by looking at your tongue in a mirror: I have noticed that the majority of my clients with digestive problems have a white or slightly green coating on their tongue. Even if you don't see a coating, if your diet is high in saturated fats, processed food or sugar, your intestines may not be as healthy as you would like them to be.

Another sign that all is not as well as it could be internally is a slight swelling or protrusion just below where the sternum ends. This could be a sign of

As we chew, enzymes in the process of breaking

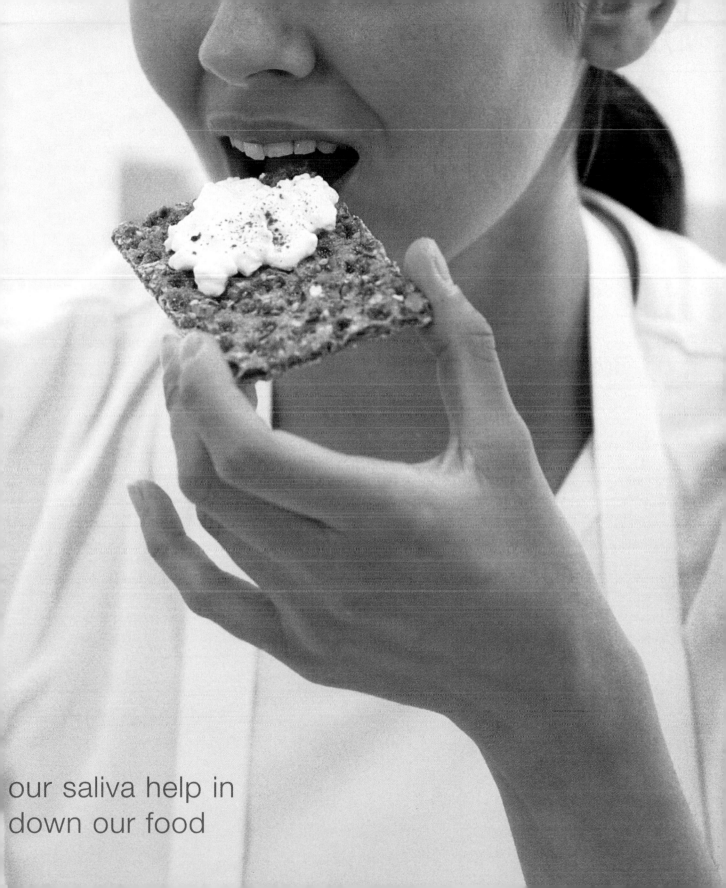

our saliva help in
down our food

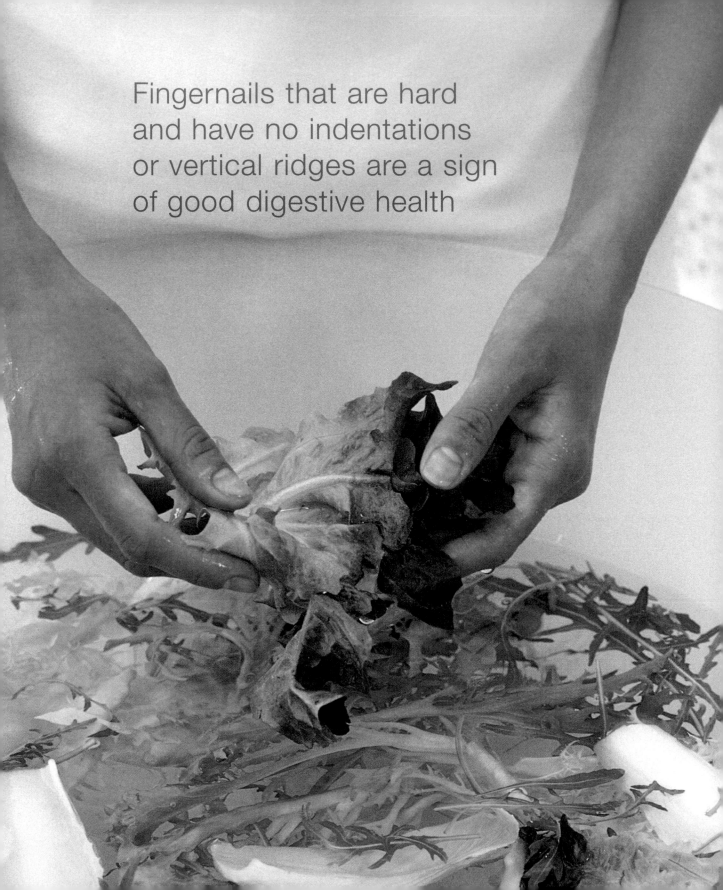

Fingernails that are hard and have no indentations or vertical ridges are a sign of good digestive health bloating. In fact, bloating is by far the most frequent complaint that I have seen in recent years. Other clues include flatulence, alternating diarrhoea and constipation and/or bad breath. Furthermore, those of my clients who have flaky or soft fingernails that break easily will often notice an improvement in the quality of their nails after appropriate changes have been made to their diet.

Hidden dangers

Beneficial bacteria are now contained in many sweetened live yoghurts and drinks, but unless you eat or drink these products in large amounts they can be limited in the extent to which they improve the levels of friendly bacteria in your system. Many products that are marketed as healthy are, in fact, loaded with sugar. This ingredient helps to make the drink palatable and, since bacteria feed on sugar, it ensures that they survive the bottling and storage process. The problem is that both friendly and unfriendly bacteria will feed on the sugar once it is in the intestines. So the health effects of these drinks or yoghurts can be limited, given their high sugar content.

Not only does sugar encourage the proliferation of unfriendly bacteria, I believe that a diet high in sugary foods can lead to weight gain and food cravings. If you exclude refined sugars from your diet, you can improve your digestive health and reduce any cravings for sugar.

You should be aware that low-fat foods are also often loaded with sugar in some form. A low-fat or calorie-controlled diet is therefore automatically higher in refined sugars than is, I believe, best for intestinal health.

High levels of yeasts

The intestines also contain yeasts that can affect digestion. The best known is *Candida albicans,* which can cause symptoms such as thrush, fatigue and sugar and alcohol cravings. Yeasts, in moderation, have a positive role to play in the intestines, but they may proliferate if your diet is high in sugar, alcohol and saturated fats.

Gut inflammation

High levels of unfriendly bacteria and yeasts and low levels of friendly bacteria can cause the intestinal lining to become inflamed. This sensitive barrier is as thin as the skin on the eyelids, so it's easy to see how vulnerable it can be. If it does become inflamed, I believe tiny food particles may pass through it, attracting the attention of the immune system which then sends out specific cells to deal with these unwanted substances. The next time you eat the same food, your immune system may react to it, even while it is still in your mouth. I consider this is how a food intolerance is born: if your gut isn't healthy and intact, today's meal can become tomorrow's problem.

Parasite problems

Parasites are the last part of the story. Transmitted on the skin or in food or water, they can cause digestive problems in the same way as unfriendly bacteria. The most common parasite is *Blastocystis hominis,* which may contribute to the condition now classified as irritable bowel syndrome (IBS).

If you suspect that you have a parasite or a bacterial problem, ask a doctor or nutrition consultant for a stool analysis, or find a good nutritional therapist to recommend an appropriate anti-parasitic herbal remedy that contains goldenseal, grapeseed extract, berberine or black walnut extract. If you are pregnant, or you are concerned about your digestive health, see a doctor first.

So, by encouraging beneficial bacteria to proliferate in the gut, and by reducing its levels of unfriendly bacteria, sugar, yeasts and any possible parasites, you can greatly improve your chances of good overall digestive health.

Eating **healthily** encourages **beneficial bacteria** to **proliferate** and **reduces** levels of potentially **unfriendly bacteria**, yeasts and any possible parasites

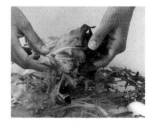

Complex and simple carbohydrates

So just what should you eat to encourage good digestive health? Foods known as carbohydrates are broken down by the body into glucose, the fuel that cells use to make energy. That's the energy necessary for every function, from breathing and thinking to moving and digesting. Carbohydrates that are low in fibre are broken down quickly into glucose to supply a surge of energy. However, your energy levels soon fall just as quickly, leaving you hungry so that you eat more food and gain weight. In contrast, carbohydrates that are high in fibre are broken down more slowly by the body. So, by eating high-fibre carbohydrates in the correct amounts, I believe that you will achieve successful weight loss.

The best way to think of food being broken down by the body is to compare, for example, a raw carrot to a glass of carrot juice. You must chew the carrot well as it's a fibrous vegetable, and it's this fibre content that slows down the rate at which the carrot is digested.

This slow conversion time ensures that the levels of glucose in the blood rise gently, so the carrot is classed as a complex carbohydrate. The fibre in the carrot has other benefits too: it helps lower cholesterol, maintains the right levels of gut bacteria and is essential for a healthy cardiovascular system; the list is almost endless.

If you take the same carrot and juice it, the nutrients may now be easier to absorb, but as the fibre has been removed the juice is broken down quickly into glucose. Despite the fact that it's rich in nutrients, the juice is effectively now a refined, or simple, carbohydrate.

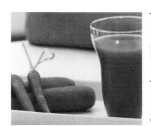

The way to think of food being **broken down** by the body is to compare a **raw carrot** to a glass of **carrot juice**

Juices and puréed soups are generally thought of as being healthy, but in my plan these foods are excluded unless they are drunk with a meal that contains protein and fibre to slow the digestion process. The high glucose levels generated by these simple carbohydrates stimulate insulin production, which can hinder weight loss.

Insulin production

Glucose levels in the blood fluctuate all the time. If levels are high and surplus to immediate requirements – that is, if glucose is not being used to create energy – the body senses this and stimulates the pancreas to release insulin. This hormone encourages the body, through a series of biochemical changes, to store excess glucose in the muscles and liver to be used later on. Once these stores are full, glucose is stored as fat. So a diet of foods that are broken down into glucose quickly will stimulate insulin production, and so add to your fat stores. If your diet only includes foods that take time to be broken down, and if you avoid large meals, your insulin levels will be kept to a minimum, allowing any fat stores to decrease.

The Food Doctor plan

By now you should have a good idea of what The Food Doctor plan is all about. In short, you will eat mainly lean proteins, essential fats, fibre and some carbohydrates, but only those that are broken down slowly.

This book begins with a seven-day diet to improve your digestion and reduce fermentation in the gut. This is the toughest part of my plan, but don't let that put you off. It's only for one week and it forms the foundation for establishing good digestive health and losing weight. You can extend this diet to two weeks if you wish, but no longer – or try it before a holiday or after Christmas.

The diet is followed by a long-term eating plan that shows you how to lose weight, slowly but surely, while benefiting from a diet rich in nutrients and fibre provided by the right balance of complex carbohydrates and proteins for good health. Remember that the success of any weight-loss plan is affected by your levels of physical activity. If you don't exercise, your chances of succeeding will be low. Following this plan with friends, family or colleagues can make things easier and provide help and support when you need it. Above all, this plan is safe, sustainable and simple. No science degree is required, no weighing of food is necessary, no food groups are excluded and, best of all, there is room to cheat too.

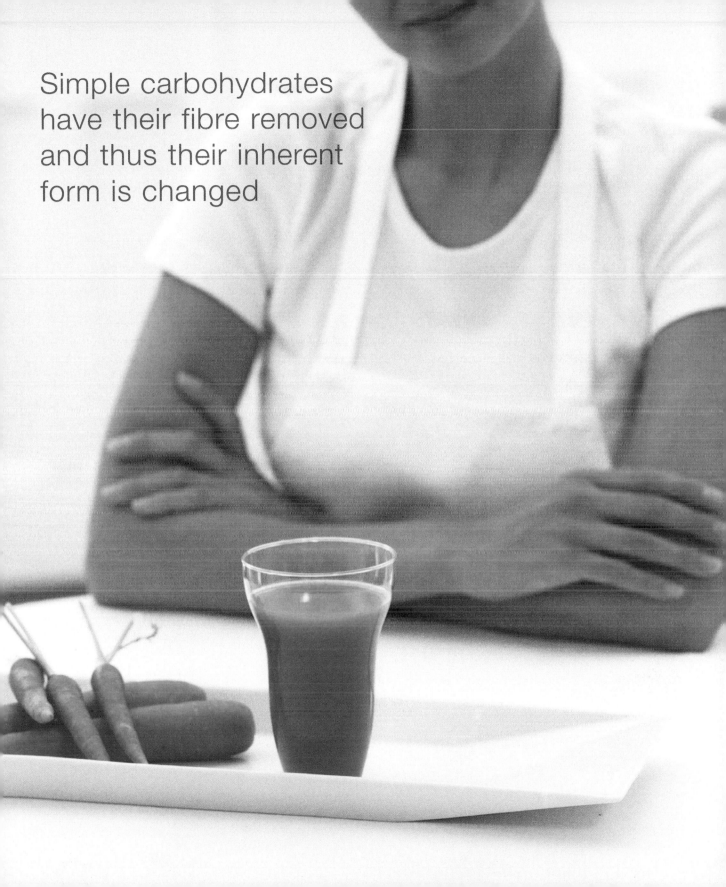

Simple carbohydrates
have their fibre removed
and thus their inherent
form is changed

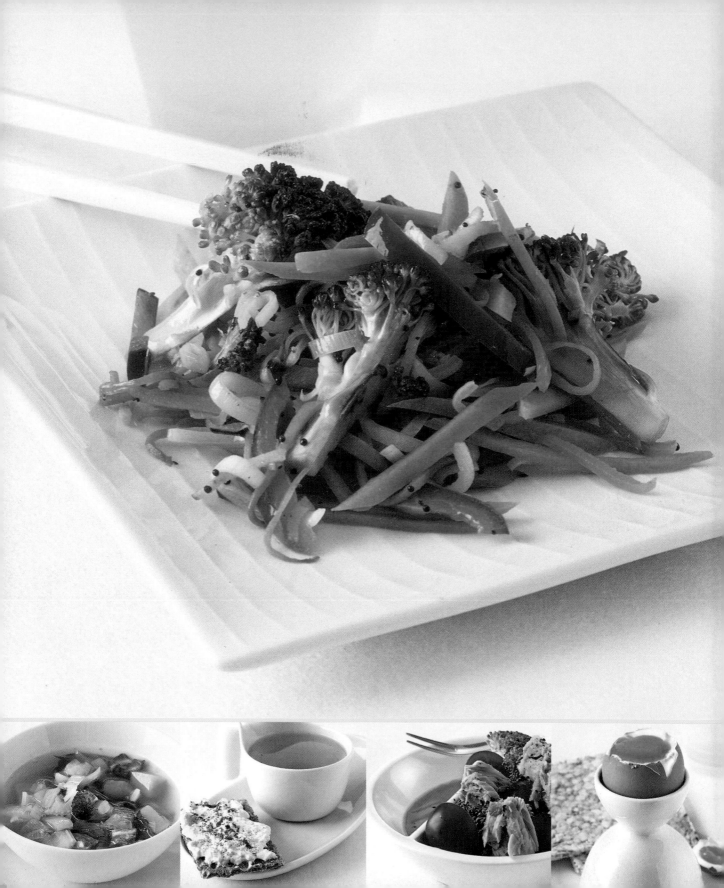

Seven-day diet

The Seven-day Diet encourages good digestive health by reducing the amount of sugars and saturated fats you eat. Seven days is sufficient for you to adapt to, and benefit from, the changes in your diet, and still achieve realistic goals. You will eat frequently, albeit in small amounts, so you shouldn't feel especially hungry. Try to stick to the suggested meals as this balanced diet plan is designed to promote health and well-being, but if there are certain foods that you would prefer not to eat, substitute one recipe for another recommended at a similar time of day. Each recipe makes one serving. Before you start, see the Note at the front of the book.

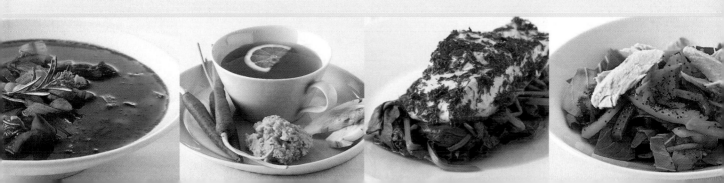

Preparing for the seven-day diet

Before you begin the Seven-day Diet, keep a food diary of what you eat and drink over three days. This will help you to identify which foods presently make up the bulk of your usual diet, and to clarify the current state of your health *(see pp.20–21)*. During this time you can shop for the ingredients you will need for the week.

Three-day diary

Before you begin the diet, the most important step is to keep a food diary. Photocopy this blank diary plan and fill it in as diligently as you can. I suggest that you write down a list of everything you eat and drink, and at what time, over three consecutive days. There is also space to write down how you feel. This could include physical symptoms – for example, whether you feel lethargic or bloated – and even, perhaps, how you feel emotionally.

The changes in your eating habits over the next week may take some getting used to, so this food diary will serve to remind you of the meals and treats you currently eat, the impact such foods have had on the state of your health and how positive the Seven-day Diet will be for your future well-being. Write yourself notes and post them in places where you keep food (the larder, fridge, your desk drawer) so that you will remember to stay resolute and not waver while you are on the diet.

DAY ONE

Time	All meals, snacks, treats and drinks

How do I feel?

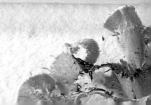

DAY TWO

Time   All meals, snacks, treats and drinks

How do I feel?

DAY THREE

Time   All meals, snacks, treats and drinks

How I feel?

Shopping for the seven-day diet

Once you decide which day you'll begin the Seven-day Diet *(see box, below)*, you can shop for most of the food you'll require before you start, leaving yourself just a few vegetables and some fresh fish to buy during the week. If you are well-stocked with all the right ingredients for the recipes, the Seven-day Diet will be much easier to follow and you will also have no excuses for straying into shops and buying unsuitable alternatives at the last minute. Photocopy the lists on these pages and tick off the ingredients as you shop for them. Buy organic food if you prefer, although the success of this diet does not depend on it.

DON'T START ON A MONDAY

How many times have you overdone things or veered from your eating plan at the weekend and then justified your actions by promising to start again on Monday? I know from experience that starting the Seven-day Diet on a Monday makes the weekend feel a long way away. I recommend starting the diet on a Wednesday or Thursday so that if you feel you need more sleep, or if you experience any of the symptoms on pages 20–21, then the weekend is just around the corner, allowing you to take things easy. By the time Monday comes around, you should be feeling good, making it easier to tackle whatever the following week holds.

Shopping list for the Seven-day Diet

Dried foods

☐ 450g (1lb) porridge oats
☐ 450g (1lb) quinoa

☐ 1 packet unsalted rice cakes
☐ 1 packet olive oil oatcakes
☐ 1 packet rye crispbreads

☐ 1 small packet pumpkin seeds
☐ 1 small packet sesame seeds
☐ 1 small packet sunflower seeds
☐ 1 small packet linseeds
☐ 1 small packet pine nuts
☐ 1 small packet cashew nuts

☐ 250g (9oz) raisins
☐ 2 small packets mixed nuts, including cashew nuts, Brazil nuts, almonds, walnuts and hazelnuts

For the muesli mix

To make the Seven-day Diet muesli mix, buy a small packet of each of any **four** of the following grains:
☐ Barley flakes
☐ Rye flakes
☐ Oat flakes
☐ Millet flakes*
☐ Rice flakes*
☐ Quinoa flakes*
☐ Buckwheat flakes*

*Choose these grains if you require a gluten-free diet.

The Seven-day Diet recipes are all simple assemblies of ingredients that require minimal preparation and cooking time.

Spices, flavourings and oils

- [ ] Cold-pressed olive oil
- [ ] Cold-pressed sesame seed oil

- [ ] Yeast-free vegetable bouillon
- [ ] Mango powder, available from spice shops or Indian food shops (or substitute with fresh lemon juice)

- [ ] 1 whole nutmeg
- [ ] 1 small jar ground cinnamon powder
- [ ] 1 small jar cardamom pods
- [ ] 1 small jar caraway seeds
- [ ] 1 small jar cumin seeds
- [ ] 1 small jar coriander seeds
- [ ] 1 small jar garam masala
- [ ] 1 small jar black peppercorns
- [ ] 1 small jar cayenne pepper
- [ ] 1 small jar tahini paste
- [ ] 1 small jar tumeric
- [ ] 1 small jar paprika

Canned foods

- [ ] 1 can mixed beans†
- [ ] 1 can lentils†
- [ ] 2 cans chick-peas†
- [ ] 2 cans chopped tomatoes†
- [ ] 2 cans tuna in spring water, unless you prefer fresh tuna

†I list canned food for simplicity. If you use dried legumes or fresh tomatoes, allow for extra soaking and cooking time. Ensure that cans contain no sugar or salt.

Fresh vegetables

- [ ] 4 medium onions
- [ ] 1 small red onion
- [ ] 1 pumpkin
- [ ] 10 carrots
- [ ] 250g (9oz) leaf spinach
- [ ] 1 small bulb Florence fennel
- [ ] 2 small or 1 large head celery
- [ ] 2 medium leeks
- [ ] 2 heads pak choi
- [ ] 4 small heads broccoli
- [ ] 1 small green cabbage

- [ ] 5cm (2in) root ginger
- [ ] 6 lemons
- [ ] 2 bulbs garlic

Salad vegetables

- [ ] 12 baby/cherry tomatoes
- [ ] 4 medium tomatoes, if not using tinned
- [ ] 1 bag mixed leaf salad
- [ ] 1 avocado
- [ ] 1 cucumber
- [ ] 3 peppers, yellow, red or orange
- [ ] 1 bunch watercress

Frozen foods

- [ ] 50g (2oz) peas
- [ ] 50g (2oz) frozen prawns, if not using fresh

Chilled foods

- [ ] 1 tub cottage cheese
- [ ] 150g (6oz) tofu
- [ ] 1 tub live natural yoghurt
- [ ] 1 tub houmous, or make your own fresh (see recipe, p.26)

- [ ] 50g (2oz) prawns if not using frozen
- [ ] 100g (4oz) white fish

- [ ] 6 free-range eggs

Fresh herbs

- [ ] Basil
- [ ] Mint
- [ ] Parsley
- [ ] Coriander
- [ ] Dill
- [ ] Rosemary
- [ ] Bay leaves
- [ ] Thyme

Food to buy during the week

- [ ] 6 medium tomatoes for day six if not using tinned tomatoes
- [ ] 300g (10oz) salmon fillet if you choose this option for dinner on day five and lunch on day six

Changes that may take place

The Seven-day Diet is designed to encourage better overall digestion by excluding the three "S"s – simple carbohydrates, stimulants and saturated fats. Since your usual diet may include some or all of these elements, it's important that you are aware of what is happening to your body during the seven days, and what these changes to your health mean.

The state of your health

Some people feel energized while they are on the Seven-day Diet, finding that they sleep well and have a clear mind. However, even if you don't feel especially good, rest assured that this programme is an important first step in achieving your goal of feeling well and eating healthily. I believe that the more of the three Ss you normally eat, the more likely you are to experience any one of the following symptoms while on the diet:

- Fatigue
- Food cravings
- Bad breath
- Mild diarrhoea
- Increased need for sleep
- Skin breakouts

Not everyone experiences unpleasant symptoms, so don't be put off by the possibility that these conditions might affect you. They are all really positive signs that things are changing for the better.

IMPORTANT PRECAUTIONS

I do not recommend that children follow any diet unless it's absolutely necessary, and then only under the supervision of an appropriate healthcare professional. No one under the age of 16 should undertake this diet plan. Likewise, do not follow this diet if you are pregnant. If you have a diagnosed medical condition, such as diabetes, please consult your doctor first.

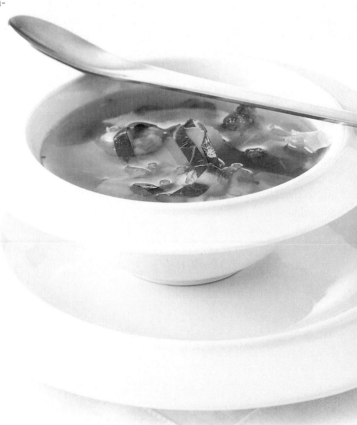

The Seven-day Diet is a short and simple programme that will help cleanse your body of the detrimental effects of the three Ss.

Signs of change

These are some of the common symptoms that you may experience during the initial stages of the Seven-day Diet, depending on how much you have previously indulged in the three Ss.

Do you feel more tired than usual?

If you have previously relied on caffeine and simple carbohydrates (see p.12) to give you short-term energy, then removing these substances from your diet will help to normalize the way your adrenal glands behave. Instead of triggering adrenaline repeatedly through the day, the adrenal glands should start to respond less often, which will keep the levels of glucose in your blood more even and help you to avoid "highs" and "lows". As this process takes place you may feel more tired than usual but don't worry, this feeling will soon pass.

Have you an increased need for sleep?

One key requirement of the Seven-day Diet is to rest, and you may notice that you have an increased need for sleep. For this reason I suggest that you don't make any plans for the week and that you stay at home whenever possible. Many people find that they sleep really deeply during the Seven-day Diet, and perhaps need more sleep than usual, so plan some early nights.

Are you craving sugary foods?

You will probably find that if you have eaten simple carbohydrates for energy in the past, you are now craving sugar and sweet foods. Such foods have encouraged the unfriendly bacteria and yeasts in your gut to proliferate (see pp.8–11), and since you are removing the simple sugars they feed on by following this diet – in effect, starving them – they can become a little demanding! If you do experience any food cravings, these should pass quickly.

Does your breath smell?

Rather than being hindered by the three Ss and processed foods, your digestive system is being encouraged to function more efficiently. As a result, you may find that you develop a green or white coating on your tongue (see p.8). This may be accompanied by bad breath. There is no need to worry as this is only a temporary symptom. Chewing parsley can help alleviate bad breath, as can cleaning your teeth and gargling with a sugar-free mouthwash.

Are you experiencing mild diarrhoea?

The increase in liquids (including water and soups) and fibre that this diet provides can stimulate bowel movements and soften the stools. This is a healthy sign, showing that the Seven-day Diet is working. Conversely, some people get slightly constipated for the first day or two but this, too, is likely to be temporary.

Have you broken out in spots?

It is possible that you may get some spots, especially around the chin area. This suggests that your digestive system is undergoing a mild cleansing. As this is a good sign that things are changing, you may have to just bear with it, and they shouldn't last long.

Seven-day diet
soups

These soups are an integral part of the Seven-day Diet for several reasons. The clear soup is a highly concentrated, cleansing drink rich in minerals. It is designed to help improve the workings of the digestive system as quickly as possible, and will also be used throughout the week to increase your fluid intake.

The other two vegetable-based soups provide your body with a high degree of easily absorbed nutrients, together with vital fibre and liquid. They will also help to promote better digestive health, which is the main aim of The Food Doctor diet.

The soups are all easy to prepare by even the most inexperienced cook, and can be stored in the fridge for up to a week, or in the freezer. Try to make these soups one day ahead of beginning the Seven-day Diet. If you work, you may like to invest in a thermos to enable you to drink these soups during the day.

Clear soup
for the 14 snacks in the Seven-day Diet

3.5 litres (6 pints) water
4 carrots, roughly chopped
½ head celery, roughly chopped
1 medium onion, quartered
2 cloves garlic, crushed
2 bay leaves
4 sprigs fresh thyme (or 1 teaspoon dried thyme)
4 whole cloves
6 black peppercorns
6 sprigs of parsley
Large handful fresh leaf spinach, coarsely shredded
Juice of 1 lemon
1 teaspoon Dijon mustard
Freshly ground black pepper, to taste
2 lemon and ginger tea bags (optional)

Put all of the ingredients, except the lemon juice, mustard, black pepper and tea bags, in a large saucepan, bring to the boil and simmer gently for 30 minutes.

Strain the liquid into a jug and throw the vegetables away. Return the broth to the pan and stir in the remaining ingredients. If using the tea bags, leave them to brew for about a minute, then lift out and discard. Store the soup in the fridge for the duration of the Seven-day Diet. The tea bags are optional but do add a freshness to the taste, and ginger is good for the digestive system.

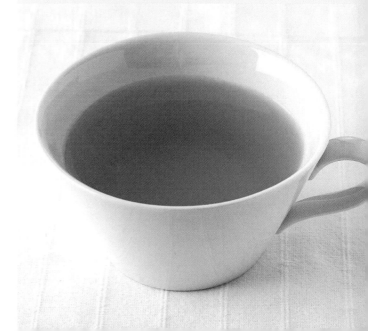

Tomato and rosemary soup

for three meals on days one, two and three

1 medium onion, diced
2 stalks celery, sliced
1 carrot, diced
1 large clove garlic, crushed
1 400g (14oz) can plum tomatoes, chopped
1 sprig fresh rosemary
1 flat teaspoon mango powder, or the juice of ½ lemon
1 litre (1¾ pints) fresh chicken or vegetable stock, or add
1 tablespoon yeast-free bouillon powder to 1 litre (1¾ pints) water
50g (2oz) shredded spinach
1 medium head pak choi, shredded

Heat two tablespoons of olive oil in a large saucepan. Add the onion, celery, carrot and garlic and cook gently over a low heat until the vegetables begin to soften. Stir in the tomatoes and add the rosemary and mango powder or lemon juice. Simmer for five minutes, then add the stock and simmer for 15 minutes or so until the vegetables are cooked but not soggy.

Stir in the spinach and pak choi and cook for two or three minutes more until they wilt. Remove the rosemary and season with freshly ground black pepper. Divide the soup into three individual portions and store in the fridge.

Chunky vegetable soup

for three meals on days four, six and seven

1 teaspoon each of caraway and cumin seeds
1 medium onion, diced
1 clove garlic, crushed
200g (7oz) pumpkin, peeled and cut into small cubes
½ small green cabbage, shredded
1 small head broccoli, broken into florets
1 stick celery, sliced
1 small carrot, diced
½ medium leek, finely sliced
1.5 litres (2½ pints) fresh chicken or vegetable stock,
or add 1½ tablespoons yeast-free bouillon powder to
1.5 litres (2½ pints) water
1 bay leaf

Put the seeds in a small, heavy-based pan and toast over a medium heat for a few minutes until lightly browned.

Gently heat two tablespoons of olive oil in a large pan and soften the onion and garlic for five minutes. Add the rest of the vegetables and the seeds. Heat them together in the oil for another five minutes or so, then add just enough stock to cover the vegetables and simmer for ten minutes. Add the remaining stock and bay leaf, season with black pepper and simmer for about 20 minutes until all the vegetables are cooked. Divide the soup into three portions and store in the fridge or freezer.

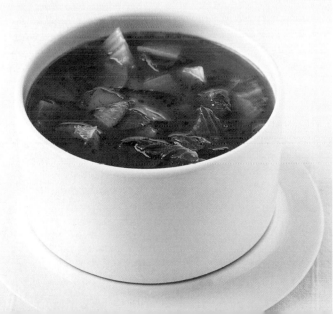

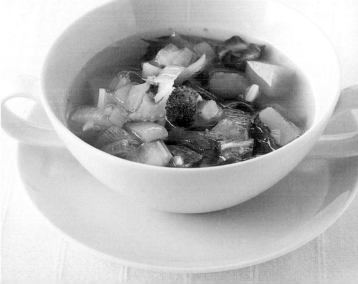

Day 1

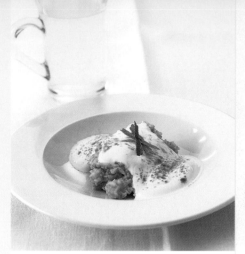

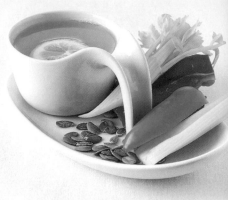

You are probably feeling full of good intentions as this is day one. In fact, this first day shouldn't prove too difficult as your food choices are tasty and varied and you won't begin to feel the effects of your change in eating habits until tonight or tomorrow morning.

Remember to drink plenty of water and herbal teas in between meals, and try to take things easy in the evening. All menus serve one.

Breakfast

This meal provides the right mix of ingredients to give your body sufficient energy and to enable you to have the best start to the day.

Glass of hot water with juice of ½ lemon

Cinnamon porridge

RECIPES

2 tablespoons porridge oats
50ml (2fl oz) water
2 tablespoons live natural yoghurt
A pinch of ground cinnamon

Combine the oats and water in a small saucepan, bring to the boil and simmer for one minute until the oats are soft.

Let the mixture stand off the heat for another minute before serving. Top with the yoghurt and a sprinkle of cinnamon.

Mid-morning snack

Your breakfast should have lasted you well into the morning but by 10.30am or so you will probably be feeling hungry enough to need this snack.

200ml (7fl oz) clear soup

2 strips each of red and orange pepper, 1 stick of celery and 1 tablespoon of pumpkin seeds

MANAGING YOUR TIME

This diet is based upon fresh, homemade meals, so you may need to allow yourself a little more time before each meal to prepare the ingredients and cook your food.

In practice, this really means getting up ten minutes earlier or so each morning to give yourself extra time to prepare your food and eat breakfast. You may even enjoy the chance to slow your pace and switch off in the evening as you prepare dinner.

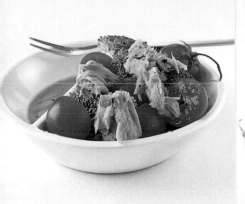

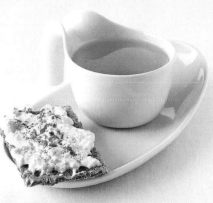

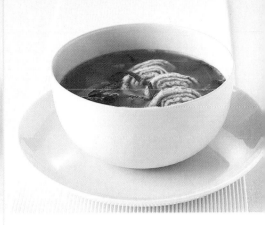

Lunch

Assuming that you ate your mid-morning snack about 10.30am, you should eat lunch around 1pm so that your energy levels stay constant.

Broccoli and tomato salad with tofu or tuna

Mid-afternoon snack

Eating in the afternoon is really important since the gap between lunch and dinner can be a long one. Aim to eat this snack around 4pm.

200ml (7fl oz) clear soup

Plain cottage cheese spread on 1 rye crispbread and topped with a pinch of garam masala

Dinner

This meal is quick and convenient if you made your soups in advance, or cook a batch of soup now *(see p.23)* and store the remainder in the fridge.

Tomato and rosemary soup with mixed beans or shredded omelette

---

Juice of ½ lemon
25g (1oz) tofu or 50g (2oz) canned tuna
50g (2oz) broccoli florets
4 cherry tomatoes, halved

Mix up a marinade of lemon juice in a small bowl and season with freshly ground black pepper.

If you are using tofu*, cut it into cubes and add it to the marinade.

If you are using tuna*, separate the flakes loosely with a fork and add them to the marinade.

Place the broccoli and tomatoes in a bowl, scatter the tofu or tuna over the top, drizzle with olive oil and serve.

*Store the remaining tofu or tuna in the fridge for lunch on day four.

MEALS TO GO

If you work in an office or are out and about most days, you may be wondering how you will manage to stick to the diet. Why not prepare your snacks and lunch the previous evening, or first thing in the morning, and store them in tupperware boxes? You can also heat your soup in the morning and bring it into work in a thermos flask.

Try to ensure that you take a break from work to eat so that the stress of the day doesn't impair your digestive process.

350ml (12½fl oz) tomato and rosemary soup
2 tablespoons mixed beans, canned or soaked and cooked, or 1 egg
A pinch of turmeric powder

If you are using mixed beans, ladle the soup into a saucepan and add the beans. Warm through over a low heat and serve.

If you are using an egg, beat it with a tablespoon of water and season with freshly ground pepper and turmeric.

Lightly oil an omelette pan using a little olive oil on a ball of kitchen roll. Pour in the egg mix and cook over a gentle heat until it sets. Flip the egg over and cook on the other side until golden. Turn it onto a wooden board, and when cool roll it up and cut into fine shreds.

Heat the soup through, stir in the shredded omelette and serve.

Day 2

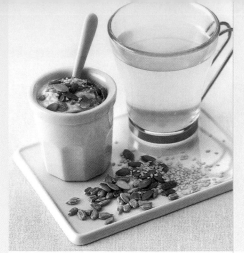

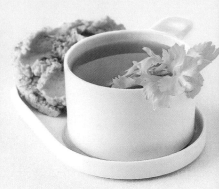

Don't give in to temptation today, since the cleansing effects of this diet are now under way, improving your digestion. Once again, ensure that you drink plenty of water, perhaps flavoured with some sliced cucumber or a squeeze of fresh lime if you need some added taste.

If this is a work day, remember to prepare your snacks and lunch to take in with you so that you can stick to the plan.

Breakfast

Ideally, you should eat within an hour of waking to replenish energy levels that have become depleted overnight. Today's breakfast is quick and easy.

Glass of hot water with juice of ½ lemon

Three-seed yoghurt

RECIPES

3 tablespoons live natural yoghurt
1 tablespoon pumpkin seeds
1 tablespoon sunflower seeds
1 heaped teaspoon sesame seeds
A pinch of ground cinnamon

Spoon three generous tablespoons of yoghurt into a bowl. Sprinkle the pumpkin, sunflower and sesame seeds over the top. Flavour with a pinch of cinnamon and serve.

Mid-morning snack

A mid-morning snack is essential to ensure that you don't feel too hungry by lunchtime. This combination will sustain you until your next meal.

200ml (7fl oz) clear soup

Houmous spread on 1 rice cake

1 420g (15oz) can chick-peas*
2 tablespoons tahini paste
2 tablespoons lemon juice
1 clove garlic, crushed
Olive oil and cayenne pepper to garnish

Blend the chick-peas, tahini, lemon juice, garlic and some freshly ground black pepper into a smooth paste in a food processor. Scrape into a small bowl, drizzle with a little olive oil and sprinkle with cayenne pepper. Cover and keep refrigerated.

Spread a rice cake with one tablespoon of the houmous for your snack.

*Save two tablespoons of chick-peas for dinner tonight if you want to add them to your soup.

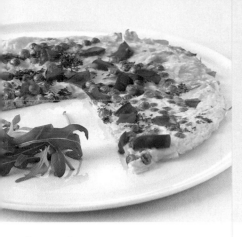

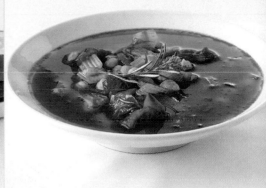

Lunch

If you made your omelette first thing this morning before going out for the day, eat it cold or reheat it if you can. Take time to chew each mouthful.

Vegetable omelette*

1 small red onion, finely chopped
1 clove garlic, crushed
2 eggs
1 tablespoon live natural yoghurt
½ teaspoon paprika
1 tablespoon chopped parsley
½ teaspoon chopped thyme
2 tablespoons peas
1 medium-ripe tomato, chopped

In a small frying pan, heat a tablespoon of olive oil over a low heat. Gently soften the onion and garlic. Beat the eggs with the yoghurt and paprika, add the herbs, season with black pepper and pour into the pan. Scatter the peas and tomato on top, cook gently until the egg sets, then turn out onto a plate and serve.

*Leave a small serving of omelette aside for your mid-afternoon snack tomorrow.

Mid-afternoon snack

Like your mid-morning snack, this combination of nuts and raw vegetables should help you to feel satisfied until dinner.

200ml (7fl oz) clear soup

10 cashew nuts, 2 thick slices of cucumber, 2 strips of pepper

WHAT CAN I DRINK?

This diet, though very short, depends on you adhering to some basic rules that will make the difference between feeling great at the end or not noticing much change at all. One important rule is to avoid alcohol, tea and coffee. This may sound like an impossible task but try it and see: you will probably find that you sleep better, wake up feeling refreshed, and experience fewer energy slumps. You should aim to drink at least eight generously sized glasses of water through the day to stay hydrated.

Dinner

All evening meals consist of protein and vegetables. You don't need to eat carbohydrates this late in the day as you will not use the energy they give.

Tomato and rosemary soup with chick-peas or flaked fish

350ml (12fl oz) tomato and rosemary soup
2 tablespoons chick-peas
or 100g (4oz) white fish fillet, cut into bite-sized pieces
Juice of ½ lemon
1 teaspoon ground coriander

If you are using chick-peas, add two tablespoons of cooked chick-peas to the soup before heating it thoroughly in a saucepan over a low heat.

If you are using fish, let it marinate in the lemon juice, ground coriander and a seasoning of freshly ground black pepper while you ladle the soup into a saucepan and heat it thoroughly. Add the fish and simmer for five minutes or until just cooked, and serve.

Day

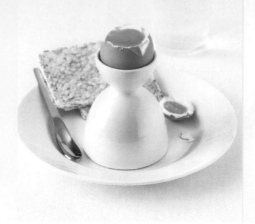

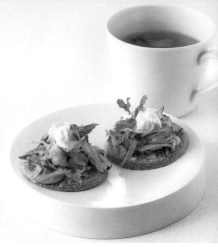

You are now nearing the halfway point of the diet, so you should be feeling a little lighter and hopefully less hungry too. Don't feel tempted to stray from the recommended foods, and take care to not overeat at mealtimes.

If you are going to be out and about today, take one portion of tomato and rosemary soup out of the fridge first thing in the morning and blend it until smooth in a processor.

Breakfast

Eggs are a great source of protein for breakfast. Boil your egg according to personal preference; the ideal time to cook a soft-boiled egg is four minutes.

Glass of hot water with juice of ½ lemon

1 boiled egg with 2 rice cakes

RECIPES

EXCLUSION ZONE

You may have noticed that the Seven-day Diet excludes any kind of meat. This is because I believe that the saturated fats in meat – and especially in red meat – promote the proliferation of unfriendly bacteria and potential yeasts in the gut *(see pp.8–11, p.50)*. These fats are detrimental to your overall digestive health in large quantities, so meat is not an option on the Seven-day Diet.

Mid-morning snack

If you work in an office, make this cucumber mint yoghurt in advance so that you can take it in to work with you and store it in a fridge.

200ml (7fl oz) clear soup

Cucumber mint yoghurt on 2 oatcakes

50g (2oz) cucumber, grated
2 tablespoons live natural yoghurt
A sprig or two of fresh mint, shredded

Mix the cucumber and yoghurt. Add the mint, season with freshly ground black pepper and mix well.

Spread on two oatcakes and serve with the soup.

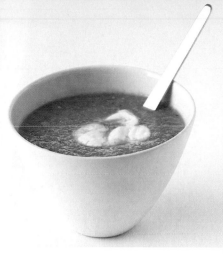

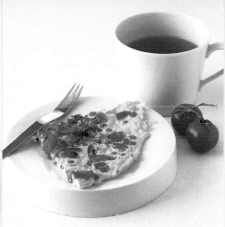

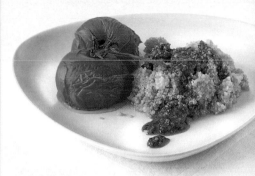

Lunch

This is the last portion of the tomato and rosemary soup, so blending it into a smooth texture will help to make it taste slightly different.

Smooth tomato and rosemary soup with yoghurt

350ml (12fl oz) tomato and rosemary soup
1 tablespoon live natural yoghurt

Blend the soup in a food processor and then heat it thoroughly in a small pan over a low heat.

Pour the hot soup into a bowl and swirl the yoghurt into it just before serving.

Mid-afternoon snack

For this instant afternoon snack, take the slice of omelette left over from yesterday lunchtime out of the fridge and eat it cold.

200ml (7fl oz) clear soup

1 small slice of omelette with 2 cherry tomatoes

FRUIT-FREE WEEK

Fruit is also off-limits on the Seven-day Diet for the simple reason that it contains a form of sugar. The natural sugar in fruit, known as fructose, can act like other sugars in the way that it encourages the growth of unfriendly bacteria and yeasts in the gut. The aim of this diet is to make your digestive system as healthy as possible, so fruit is off the menu for the duration of these seven days only.

Dinner

This meal is very nutritious and will take you about 25 minutes to cook. Remember to save a spoonful of pesto for tomorrow morning's snack*.

Quinoa with pesto and roast tomatoes

2 medium tomatoes
2 sprigs fresh rosemary
For the pesto:
  1 large handful fresh basil
  100ml (3½fl oz) olive oil
  100g (4oz) pine nuts
  1 small clove garlic
50g (2oz) quinoa
100ml (3½fl oz) water with ½ teaspoon of yeast-free bouillon powder added

Preheat the oven to 200°C/400°F/Gas 6.

Put the tomatoes and rosemary in a baking dish, drizzle with olive oil and roast for 20 minutes. Meanwhile, blend the pesto ingredients in a processor. Simmer the quinoa and water in a pan until soft, stir in three teaspoons of pesto and serve with the tomatoes (remove the rosemary sprigs first).
*Store the remaining pesto in the fridge.

Day 4

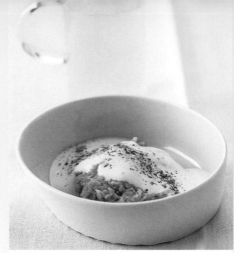

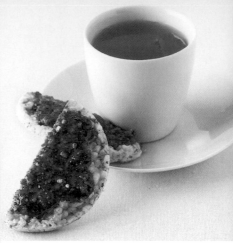

Today you will continue to eat lightly, so try to make sure that you are busy doing something that you enjoy in order to keep yourself occupied.

If you have already cooked and frozen the chunky vegetable soup, take a portion out of the freezer first thing in the morning and let it defrost in the fridge during the day, ready for dinner. Try to rest in the evening and have an early night if you need to.

Breakfast

The oats in porridge aid the efficient functioning of your digestive system and provide much-needed energy to get you through the morning.

**Glass of hot water
with juice of ½ lemon**

Nutmeg porridge

RECIPES

2 tablespoons porridge oats
50ml (2fl oz) water
2 tablespoons live natural yoghurt
Freshly grated nutmeg

Combine the oats and water in a small saucepan, bring to the boil and simmer for one minute until the oats are soft.

Let the mixture stand off the heat for another minute, then add the yoghurt and nutmeg and serve.

Mid-morning snack

Use the remaining pesto left over from last night's meal for this snack. Squeeze a little lemon juice over the top if you want to lift the flavours.

200ml (7fl oz) clear soup

Pesto spread on 1 rice cake

Spread a rice cake with a generous helping of pesto to eat with your soup.

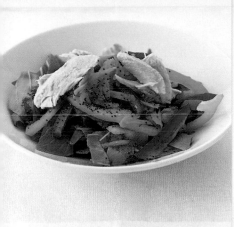
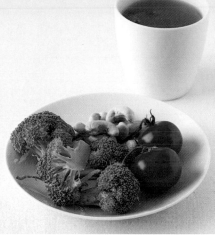
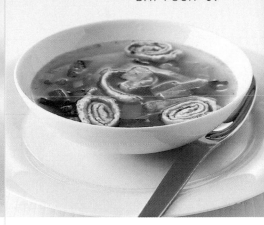

Lunch

Try to take time to sit down and eat your lunch slowly without any stress. Chewing thoroughly will also enable you to digest your food properly.

Pepper and pak choi salad with tuna or tofu

Mid-afternoon snack

This energizing snack will help you to avoid the mid-afternoon slump in energy that often follows after lunch or a busy morning's work.

200ml (7fl oz) clear soup

10 cashew nuts, 5 small florets of broccoli and 2 cherry tomatoes

Dinner

Try not to eat dinner too late in the evening. You should allow for a minimum of at least two hours in between eating and going to bed.

Chunky vegetable soup with mixed beans or shredded omelette

Juice of ½ lemon
A pinch of garam masala
25g (1oz) tofu, cut into bite-sized pieces, or 50g (2oz) canned tuna from day one
½ red or yellow pepper, cut into strips
1 small head pak choi, shredded
1 tablespoon grated carrot

Combine the lemon juice and garam masala in a small bowl and season with freshly ground black pepper. Add the tofu or tuna to this marinade and leave to one side for a few minutes.

Put the pepper and pak choi in a salad bowl and toss in a dressing of olive oil and freshly ground black pepper. Top with the carrot, spoon over the tuna or tofu with its marinade and then serve.

SHOP FOR THE NEXT FEW MEALS

Look ahead now to tomorrow's menu to make sure that you have all the ingredients you will require.

You'll need to buy some fresh salmon today or tomorrow if you intend to have this option for your evening meal on day five. You may also need to buy a few extra vegetables and some more live natural yoghurt if you have used up these ingredients.

350ml (12½fl oz) chunky vegetable soup
2 tablespoons mixed beans, canned or soaked and cooked, or 1 egg
A pinch of turmeric powder

If you are using mixed beans, ladle the soup into a saucepan and add the beans. Warm through over a low heat and serve.

If you are using an egg, beat it with a tablespoon of water and season with freshly ground pepper and turmeric.

Lightly oil an omelette pan using a little olive oil on a ball of kitchen roll. Pour in the egg mix and cook over a gentle heat until it sets. Flip the egg over and cook on the other side until golden. Turn it onto a wooden board, and when cool roll it up and cut into fine shreds.

Heat the soup through, stir in the shredded omelette and serve.

Day 5

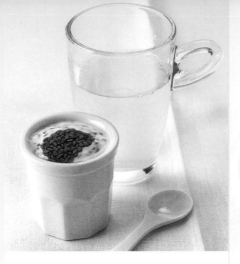
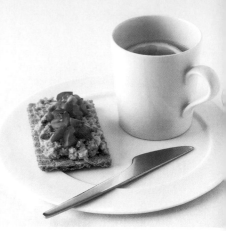

You are now over the halfway point, and your body is responding to the different elements in your diet. You may also notice some of the physical changes that are described on pages 20–21.

There are only three more days to go, so resist giving in to any temptation at this stage of the diet. If it is the weekend, keep yourself busy with an activity that you enjoy and concentrate on the sense of well-being you might now be feeling.

Breakfast

Linseeds encourage regular bowel movements and provide essential nutrients. You will need to chew the linseeds well to break them up.

Glass of hot water with juice of ½ lemon

Soaked linseeds with natural yoghurt

RECIPES

1 tablespoon linseeds
3 tablespoons live natural yoghurt
A pinch of ground cinnamon

Soak the linseeds overnight in enough water to just cover them.

In the morning drain the water away and combine the seeds with the yoghurt. Serve with a sprinkle of cinnamon on top.

Mid-morning snack

If you need to make this snack in advance, squeeze plenty of lemon juice over the avocado to prevent it going brown and store it in the fridge.

200ml (7fl oz) clear soup

Avocado spread on 1 rye crispbread with chopped tomato

½ small avocado
A good squeeze of lemon juice
1 cherry tomato, chopped

Combine the avocado, lemon juice and a seasoning of freshly ground black pepper in a bowl and mash together with a fork.

Spread the mixture on the rye crispbread, scatter the chopped tomato over the top and serve with the soup.

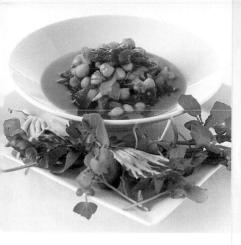
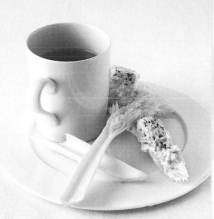
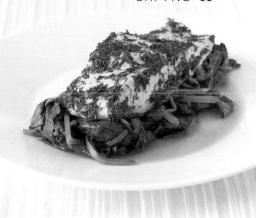

Lunch

Don't increase the portion size of this recipe according to how hungry you think you might be. The serving listed here is designed to satisfy you.

Quick chick-pea stew

Mid-afternoon snack

Eating this snack at about the same time each day enables your energy levels to stay even so that you don't feel tempted to stray from the diet.

200ml (7fl oz) clear soup
Tuna dip with celery or carrot sticks

Dinner

Don't forget to save a spoonful of spinach and a small portion of salmon for tomorrow. Alternatively, you may prefer a poached egg with the spinach.

Spinach with herb salmon or a poached egg

½ teaspoon cumin seeds
2 cardamom pods
1 medium onion, chopped
2 cloves garlic, crushed
400g (14oz) ripe or canned tomatoes, chopped
1 420g (15oz) can chick-peas
475ml (17fl oz) water

Gently heat a tablespoon of olive oil in a medium-sized saucepan, add the spices and cook for one minute. Add the onion and garlic, soften for five minutes, then stir in the tomatoes and chick-peas. Pour in the water and simmer for 10–15 minutes, stirring occasionally, until the sauce thickens.

Serve two tablespoons of stew with a salad dressed with olive oil and lemon juice. Refrigerate the remaining stew.

20g (1oz) canned tuna
2 tablespoons live natural yoghurt
A few sprigs of fresh parsley, chopped
A pinch of cayenne pepper

Mash the tuna with the yoghurt, season with freshly ground black pepper and stir in the chopped parsley.

Scoop up the dip with celery, chopped carrot sticks or Florence fennel and sprinkle a little cayenne pepper on top before serving with the soup.

300g (10oz) salmon fillet or 1 egg
A handful of chopped dill, coriander, parsley
Juice of ¼ lemon
1 clove of garlic, finely chopped
100g (4oz) fresh leaf spinach, washed
A pinch of garam masala

If you are using salmon, preheat the oven to 180°C/350°F/Gas 4. Coat the fish in the herbs, place on an oiled sheet of foil and season with lemon juice, black pepper and garlic. Fold the ends of the foil into a parcel. Cook for 20 minutes.

If you are using an egg, poach it in a frying pan of boiling water until it is set.

Put the spinach in a medium saucepan and cook over a gentle heat until wilted. Drain well. Drizzle with a little sesame seed oil, lemon juice and garam masala. Top with the salmon or egg and serve.

Day 6

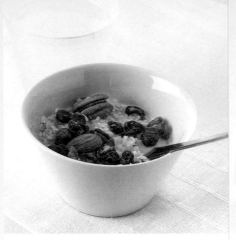

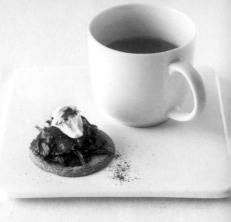

You are almost there, so persevere for these last two days and you will soon be reaping the benefits.

If you have frozen your home-made soup, then take the last two portions out of the freezer first thing this morning and let them defrost in the fridge over the course of the day.

Take things easy if you are tired, although some people can feel quite energized by this stage.

Breakfast

If you are following a gluten-free diet, make sure you choose those grains marked with an asterisk* when you mix up your muesli.

Glass of hot water with juice of ½ lemon

Muesli with whole milk or natural yoghurt

RECIPES

Choose 1 tablespoon each from any **four** of the following grains:
  Barley flakes
  Rye flakes
  Oat flakes
  Millet flakes*
  Rice flakes*
  Quinoa flakes*
  Buckwheat flakes*
8–9 mixed nuts, including hazelnuts, Brazil nuts, cashew nuts, almonds, walnuts
1 teaspoon raisins

Combine the dried ingredients in a bowl, add one tablespoon of live natural yoghurt or your choice of milk (either whole cows', goats' or sheep's milk or an unsweetened substitute such as rice or soya milk) and serve.

Mid-morning snack

Use the extra spoonful of spinach from last night's meal for this snack. Squeeze over a little lemon juice if you want to lift the flavours slightly.

200ml (7fl oz) clear soup

Spinach and yoghurt on 1 oatcake

Chop the spinach and spread it on one oatcake. Top with a teaspoon of yoghurt and sprinkle over a little cayenne pepper before serving with the soup.

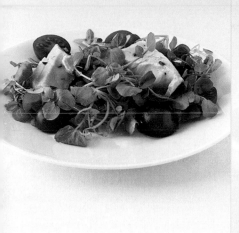
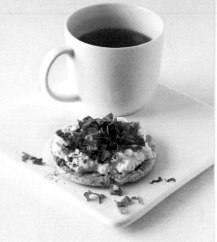
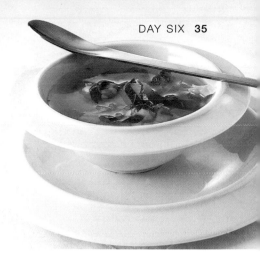

Lunch

If you had salmon for dinner last night, then use the remaining fish in this salad. If you had a poached egg, slice up an avocado instead.

Avocado or cold salmon with watercress salad

Mid-afternoon snack

Any cravings you may have had for sweet, sugary food will hopefully have passed by now, so you should enjoy this sustaining snack.

200ml (7fl oz) clear soup

Cottage cheese spread on 1 rice cake, topped with chopped fresh coriander

Dinner

Add either a spoonful of yesterday's quick chick-pea stew to tonight's soup or include a few cooked prawns instead if you prefer.

Chunky vegetable soup with chick-peas or prawns

⅛ teaspoon of cumin seeds
A handful of fresh watercress, rocket, lambs lettuce or other green salad leaves
A squeeze of lemon juice
4 cherry tomatoes, halved
½ avocado, sliced, or cold salmon

Toast the cumin seeds gently in a small heavy-based saucepan for one minute, then remove from the heat.

Dress the salad leaves with the dry-roasted cumin seeds, lemon juice, a drizzle of olive oil and freshly ground black pepper. Add the tomatoes, mix well and serve with the salmon or avocado.

EXERCISE

It is fine to exercise while you are on the Seven-day Diet, although don't overdo things and make sure you can rest for a while afterwards. You may want to time your exercise to fit in before a snack or a meal so that you can refuel quickly and not feel overly hungry.

Don't attempt any unfamiliar sports or training sessions while on this diet, since this may exhaust you or prove to be too excessive.

300ml (10fl oz) chunky vegetable soup
50g (2oz) cooked prawns
or 1 tablespoon quick chick-pea stew

Pour the soup into a saucepan and add the prawns or the chick-pea stew. Heat thoroughly over a low heat and serve.

Day 7

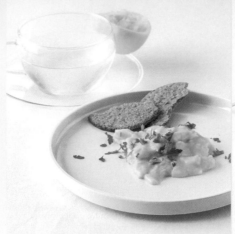

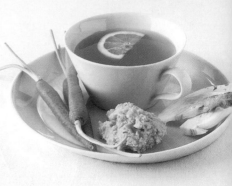

Well done, it's your last day. I hope that you didn't find the diet too difficult to follow and that by now you are feeling well, more energized and inspired to move on to the next stage, the Plan for Life *(see pp.38–91).*

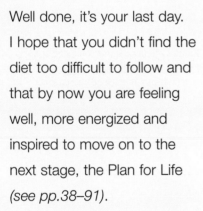

Breakfast

Try to continue the routine of preparing a nutritious, well-balanced breakfast of protein and carbohydrate such as this after you finish the diet.

**Glass of hot water
with juice of ½ lemon
Scrambled egg with 1 oatcake**

RECIPES

1 egg
1 teaspoon live natural yoghurt
A pinch of turmeric powder
1 tablespoon fresh parsley, chopped
1 oatcake

Beat together the egg and the yoghurt, then season with freshly ground black pepper and add a pinch of ground turmeric powder.

Heat a little olive oil in a small saucepan, pour in the beaten egg and cook over a low heat until the egg forms soft curds. Once cooked, stir in the parsley and serve with one oatcake.

Mid-morning snack

If you made your own houmous on day two, you can use up the rest of it for this snack. Otherwise use some shop-bought houmous.

**200ml (7fl oz) clear soup
1 tablespoon of houmous
with raw vegetables**

1 tablespoon houmous
A small selection of raw vegetables such as carrots, Florence fennel or celery, sliced

Serve the dip and crudités with the soup, using the vegetables to scoop up the houmous.

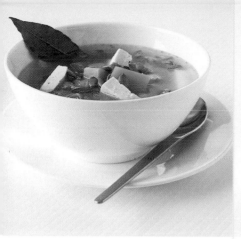
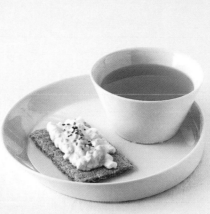
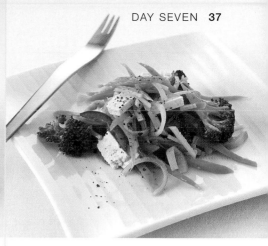

Lunch

Add a few pieces of tofu or some pumpkin seeds to this final serving of your homemade soup in order to vary the taste slightly.

Chunky vegetable soup with tofu or pumpkin seeds

Mid-afternoon snack

This is the last of the nutrient-rich clear soup that has helped to cleanse and improve your digestive system and kept your fluid intake high.

200ml (7fl oz) clear soup

Cottage cheese spread on 1 rye crispbread

Dinner

Use up the remaining vegetables in your fridge for this stir-fry and add some pumpkin seeds or the remaining tofu that you saved from lunchtime.

Stir-fried vegetables with marinated tofu or pumpkin seeds

350ml (12fl oz) chunky vegetable soup
50g (2oz) tofu*, finely cubed,
or 1 heaped teaspoon pumpkin seeds

Pour the soup into a saucepan and warm it up gently over a low heat. Add the tofu or pumpkin seeds, transfer to a bowl and serve.

*Store the rest of the tofu in the fridge for tonight's supper.

THE BENEFITS OF THE SEVEN-DAY DIET

As you come to the end of the Seven-day Diet you should hopefully feel some or all of the following:

- Improved digestion, and therefore enhanced absorption of nutrients
- Sense of well-being
- More energy
- Reduced sugar cravings
- Reduced cravings for caffeine and alcohol.

Approx.150g (5½oz) various vegetables such as carrot, pepper, leek, broccoli
2 tablespoons lemon juice
½ teaspoon fresh ginger, grated
2 cardamom seeds, ground *(see p.129)*
50g (2oz) tofu, finely cubed,
or 1 heaped teaspoon pumpkin seeds

Slice the vegetables finely. Mix the lemon juice, ginger and cardamom seeds in a bowl and season with freshly ground black pepper. If you are using tofu, toss the vegetables and tofu in this marinade. Leave to stand for 15 minutes.

Heat a tablespoon of water in a wok, add the vegetables and cook them quickly over a high heat until they are cooked but crisp. Drizzle with cold-pressed sesame seed oil. If you are using pumpkin seeds, sprinkle them over just before serving.

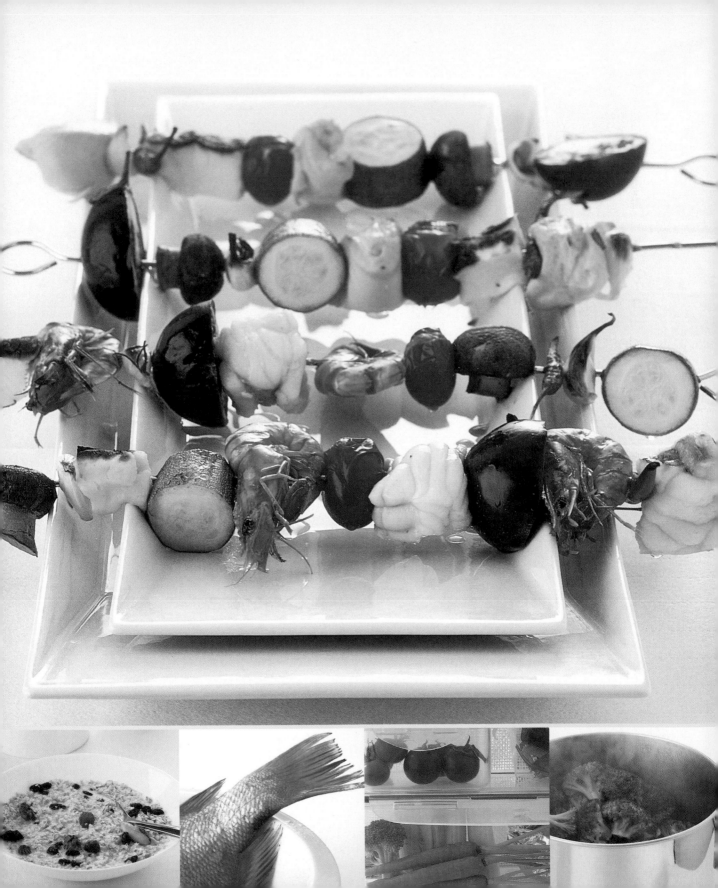

Plan for life

The Plan for Life is a simple, sustainable eating programme that is designed to be adapted to your individual lifestyle. It is important that you read through this whole section before starting so that you understand and become familiar with the ten basic Food Doctor principles – the essential guidelines on how to eat for health and well-being. Once you begin to incorporate the principles into your own routines you may want to plan ahead a little to ensure you have the appropriate foods for the right meals, but hopefully this plan will soon become second nature to you.

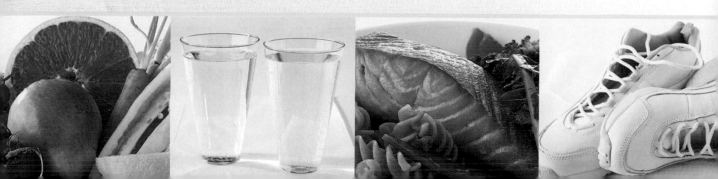

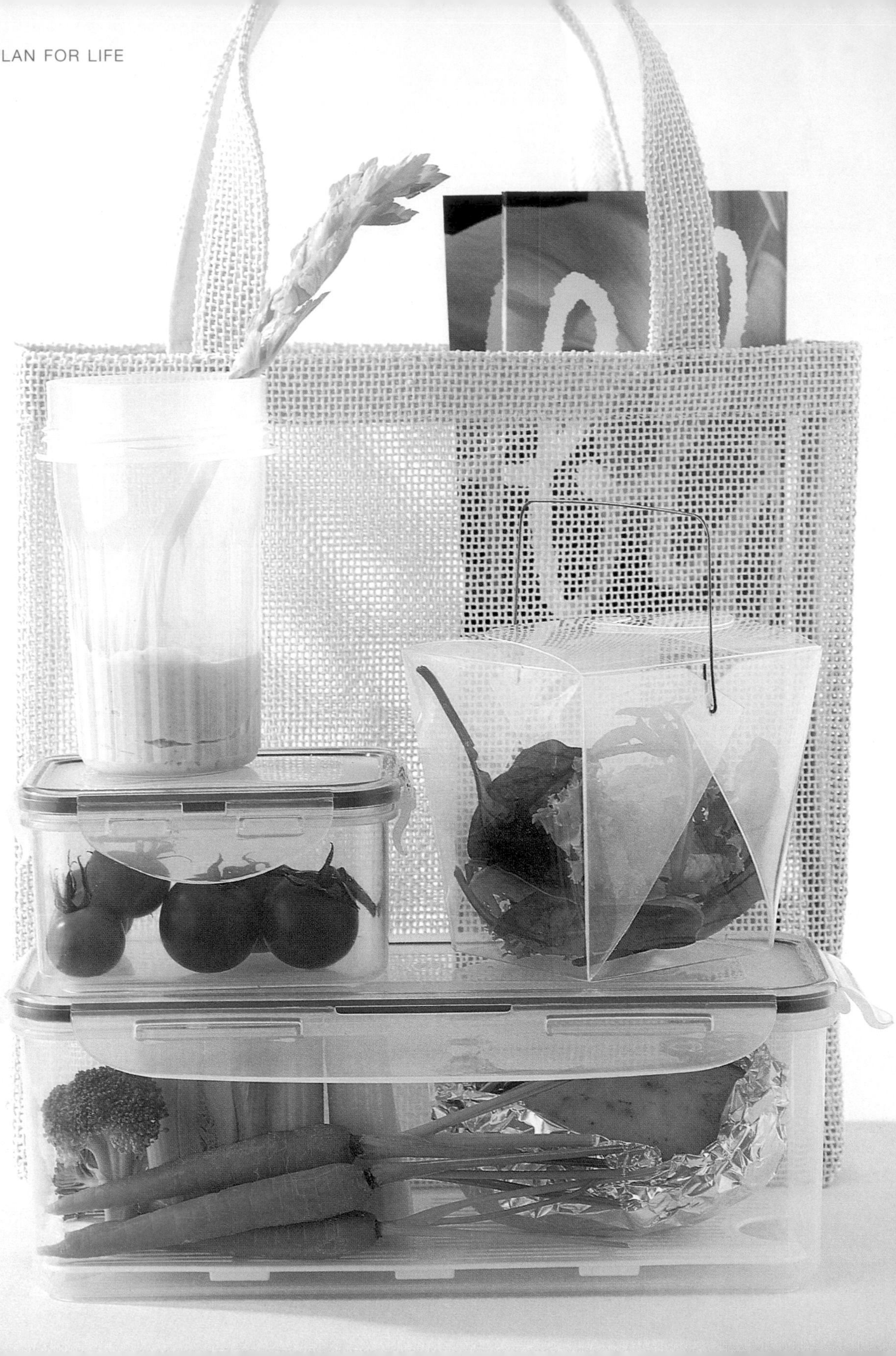

Eating for life

Any diet plan should be a sensible one that incorporates all the best that food can offer, from nutrients and fibre to flavour and taste. I believe that the process of safe, sustainable weight loss and healthy eating advocated by the Plan for Life will help you to look and feel your best.

While the Seven-day Diet is primarily designed to encourage good digestive health, the Plan for Life shows you how to eat well with plenty of choice, how to lose weight steadily and yet still be able to enjoy special occasions and have a social life. It even allows you to veer away from time to time to enjoy your favourite treat.

The following pages reveal ten crucial Food Doctor principles and explain how and why changes in your diet may need to be made, and what you can expect as a result of those changes. The principles cover several areas, including how to combine foods effectively, what to drink, when to eat for maximum energy and how to avoid hunger. I am confident that this set of principles will provide a really solid base for you to apply to your own lifestyle so that you develop great eating habits.

Plan of action

It may be that some of these principles are familiar to you, or that a few of them are already a part of your daily life, but it is important that you incorporate all the principles as a whole if you want to reap the optimum benefits. I suggest that you read right through this section first before introducing each principle, one at a time, over a period of weeks. Thus, during week one you can make changes in line with Principle 1, then after a few days introduce Principle 2, and so on. Within a month you will find that you have made some real changes, but don't rush it or you will set yourself up to fail. I have seen too many diets falter and good intentions fly out of the window because people set unrealistic goals that make the whole process daunting.

If you feel that you have a lot of weight to lose, then aim to lose a few pounds each month, which is, after all, how you gained the weight in the first place. Similarly, if you want to shed only a few pounds then that, too, should be undertaken slowly. You probably know from experience that fast weight-loss is unsustainable; if you do manage to lose weight then you will inevitably gain it – and more – back again before too long.

By sticking to the Plan for Life 100 per cent of the time and exercising regularly, you'll achieve maximum weight loss. However, if this approach proves hard to sustain, why not think of this plan as a life-changing experience that will improve your health and self-image while still giving you a chance to eat what you like once in a while (see pp.68–69)?

The Plan for Life should suit almost every lifestyle. It has been designed to reduce your levels of hunger, it's easy to follow and you don't have to buy obscure foods. Remember, too, that packaged and convenience foods are often far higher in sugar and saturated fats than any meals you make at home. However convenient they may be, they are for emergencies only, not for every day.

WHAT IF I'M PREGNANT?

I do not recommend dieting if you are pregnant as weight gain associated with pregnancy is a natural and important process. However, The Food Doctor plan is a plan for life so you can follow it at any time, even if you are pregnant or breast-feeding. Do not watch your weight, just eat well. By ensuring that you eat fresh foods, you cook for yourself when you can and you avoid stimulants and processed foods, you should find that you won't gain excess weight, only what is natural during pregnancy. There is plenty of time to lose weight after your baby is born.

Good shopping habits

Unless you are lucky enough to live near a wonderful food market, shopping for food isn't always guaranteed to be the most enthralling pastime. Yet if you allow for a little extra time when you next shop, you may be tempted by a whole range of healthy, delicious foods you haven't noticed before.

With time now at such a premium, most of us consider food shopping to be a time-consuming, repetitive chore that prevents us doing something else supposedly more worthwhile. It's all too easy to assume that it is not worth spending our precious time on the process of shopping, cooking and eating.

Ever-increasing sales of ready-made foods tend to reflect this growing attitude, and yet the sort of food I believe we should all be eating doesn't come packaged in boxes with microwaving instructions. It's likely that if you have gained weight in the past you will be familiar with these types of processed meals. The truth is that a basic homemade meal takes far less time to prepare than you might think, and it invariably tastes much more delicious than ready-made food *(see box, below)*.

Change your shopping habits
Try this simple test at home. Make a list of all the foods you usually buy, including treats, low-fat alternatives, canned drinks and ready-made meals, and file it away. Then take a look at the recommended carbohydrates and proteins for the Plan for Life *(see pp.50–53)* and make a new shopping list for yourself using those charts as a template. You will see that the foods listed are familiar and require no special trips to obscure, out-of-the-way

---

MAKE YOUR OWN CONVENIENCE FOOD

Homemade soup is a great example of a convenient, healthy meal that can be frozen and then thawed quickly *(see pp.123–24)*. After all, what could be more instant than warming some soup quickly and adding a can of beans and some fresh herbs? A delicious, easy meal with a good balance of carbohydrates, fibre and protein.

---

shops. Your supermarket probably stocks all of these foods, yet for one reason or another they haven't caught your attention before. As you shop, familiarize yourself with these different products and stock up with them for your new eating plan.

Should I buy organic food?
In the same way that the term "low fat" has come to imply "healthy", labelling food as organic can suggest added benefits. Organic fruit and vegetables are generally more expensive that non-organic alternatives and if you can afford them, or choose to make them part of your shopping list, go ahead and buy them. However, the organic nature of fruit and vegetables isn't going to make a significant difference to the success of this plan. Since so many of us fail to eat the recommended five portions of fruits and vegetables a day, it's better to eat five non-organic varieties than two or three organic ones.

When it comes to poultry, meat and fish, however, I do believe that there is a difference. These foods have been devalued, and we expect not to have to pay that much for them. Organic meat is produced using traditional methods of raising animals, hence the higher cost – and better flavour. While an organic chicken may be twice as expensive as a battery-raised one, the flavour alone is worth the extra money. You are likely to value it far more and enjoy eating it as well.

Cheaper meat, unlike organic meat, is not guaranteed to be free of chemical residues, antibiotics and hormones, so it's no wonder that the flavour might not be exciting. It also means that you probably add breadcrumbs, fatty sauces or side dishes to make the meal more interesting.

So bear in mind that shopping for quality foods encourages a healthier relationship with eating, potentially giving you a clearer palate that allows you to taste and enjoy all the ingredients in your meals.

Which is best?

Convenience food

I have noticed that many people who battle with their weight eat more ready-made meals than fresh, homemade food. The levels of sugars and fats in these meals are a large part of the problem. By all means keep a few ready-made meals in the freezer for emergencies, but only eat them occasionally when you really have no other choice.

Canned food

I have no problem with canned food: it's cheap, easy to store and convenient for meals and snacks, but do ensure that you buy products that contain no added sugar or salt. Cans of conventional baked beans, for example, tend to contain far more sugar than you might imagine, so look out for varieties that are free of sugar or that are sweetened with a little apple juice instead. It's also worth having some cans of vegetables in your store cupboard but, again, avoid any salted or sugared products.

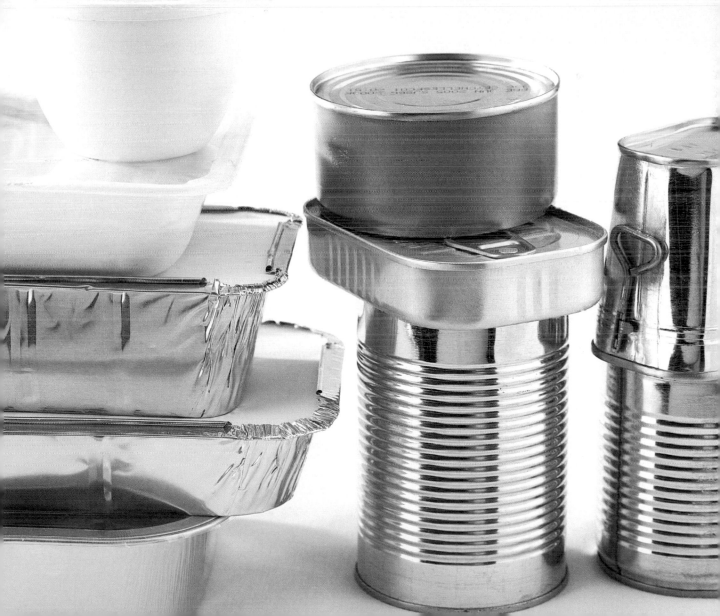

Cooking techniques

If you don't consider yourself to be adept in the kitchen, or if you find preparing and cooking food a laborious and boring chore, then it's time to consider how this issue may have contributed to your weight gain. Cooking can be an easy, even enjoyable, pastime.

The plethora of cookery shows and celebrity chefs on television these days is a good indicator of just how much we love cooking – or at least love watching other people do it. I find that every time I watch one of these shows it almost puts me off cooking, as I feel I can't attain the chefs' high standards. However, cooking needn't be complicated and you need fewer ingredients than you might imagine to make a tasty meal. Try the recipes at the back of this book (see pp.104–37) and you will find that they are easy to follow and do not take much time to prepare. And I am sure that once the ten principles of the Plan for Life (see pp.46–73) have become second nature to you, you will be happy to apply them to preparing and cooking your own food.

Steaming fish and vegetables

Ideally, all vegetables should be lightly steamed rather than boiled so that the fibre of the vegetables remains mostly intact. I suggest that when you steam vegetables you do so for just a few minutes – less than you might imagine. The colours and flavours of steamed vegetables are also far more appetising than those that are boiled and overcooked. So investing in a microwave steamer or hob steamer, or even a steamer basket that you just pop over a pan of water, is a wise move.

The good fats in fish are affected by very high temperatures, so steaming is actually a perfect way to cook most fish. It's fast too – it often takes no more than ten minutes to achieve a perfectly cooked piece of fish.

Poaching in water

Poaching fish or chicken in a pan of water is really very easy, and it is another excellent way of retaining flavour, colour and texture. You can add herbs or stock cubes to the cooking water for added flavour. Be vigilant if you use this method as poached food can easily over-cook.

Grilling and roasting

It is all too easy for the essential fats and fibre in food to be impaired if the temperature of your oven or grill is set too high. If you roast or grill your food on a medium-to-low heat, you will preserve the nutrients and still enjoy delicious results.

Why can't I fry food?

The worst way to cook food is to fry it. The very high temperatures needed for frying affects the quality of essential fats in food and converts the oil you cook with from a stable "good" fat into an unstable "bad" fat. This increases the levels of free radicals – substances that are believed to be involved in the initiation of heart disease and cancer. Your fat intake will also be higher than it need be as frying encourages food to absorb much of the fat in which it has been cooked. I strongly recommend that you avoid eating fried food in restaurants because of the unusually high quantities of fats most chefs use to enhance the flavours. If you are going to fry food, buy a wok and learn how to stir-fry: move the ingredients quickly round the wok and use just a little sunflower oil to cook with. By keeping your cooking methods as fat-free as possible your meals will be much healthier.

KEEP IT SIMPLE

Cooking needn't be complicated, so I always suggest to people who are reluctant to cook that they try to keep it simple. The principles of the Plan for Life work just as well with a piece of grilled fish and some steamed vegetables or a bowl of soup and wholemeal bread as they do with a more complicated meal containing several courses.

Why is steaming best?

The valuable nutrients in fresh food aren't affected too much by steaming, and the fibre content of vegetables is left mostly intact. Since fibre is vital for maintaining a healthy digestive system, steaming is my preferred and recommended method of cooking to promote optimum digestive health.

Principle 1
Eat protein with complex carbohydrates

The first Food Doctor principle is based on the fact that some foods are converted into glucose quickly while other foods take longer to be broken down. By understanding how to combine the right foods in the correct proportions, you will remain full of energy and still be able to lose weight.

Understanding the speed at which different foods are broken down into glucose for the body to use as fuel is crucial to The Food Doctor plan. Simple carbohydrates are quickly converted into glucose once they are digested, while protein and complex carbohydrates take longer to be broken down. The glycaemic index (GI) is a measure of how high blood-glucose levels rise after different foods have been digested. So if you eat only foods that have a slow conversion rate – in other words, a low GI score (*see pp.50–53*) – your body receives a steady supply of energy and prevents excess glucose being stored as fat.

Rather than having to remember the individual GI value of every food, there is an easier way to follow this principle. If you learn to combine the right proportions of protein and fibrous vegetables for every meal and snack, then this plan should work for you. The best way to begin to understand this concept is to look at the food on your plate and ask yourself, "Where is the protein?"

Complete proteins

Proteins contain amino acids, which are, in effect, the building blocks of the body. There are 22 amino acids in total, of which eight are classed as essential for adults (*see p.138*) as they cannot be generated by the body and must come from your diet. These essential amino acids, known as complete proteins, contain all the elements the body needs to generate the remaining amino acids. Examples of complete proteins are fish, tofu and eggs.

THE FOOD DOCTOR EQUATION

ANIMAL OR VEGETABLE
COMPLETE PROTEIN

STARCHY OR VEGETABLE
COMPLEX CARBOHYDRATES

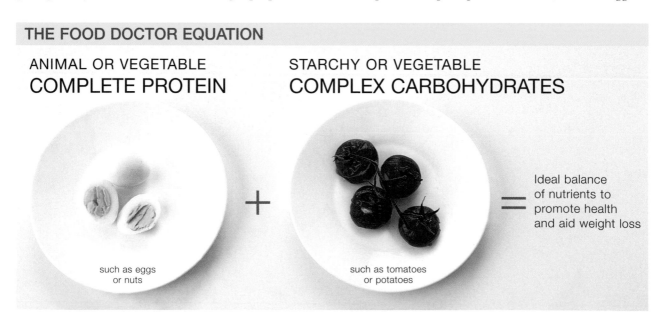

such as eggs
or nuts

such as tomatoes
or potatoes

Ideal balance
of nutrients to
promote health
and aid weight loss

The right combination?

protein 0%

complex carbohydrates 90%
of which starch 80%, vegetables 10%

simple carbohydrates 0%

vegetable fat 10%

low in fibre

Wholewheat pasta with tomato sauce

Although this meal looks healthy, there is no source of protein and the fibre content is low. The proportion of vegetable carbohydrates to starchy carbohydrates in the form of wholewheat pasta is also far too low.

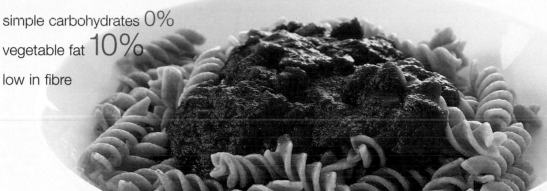

fast

glucose conversion

protein 40%

complex carbohydrates 50%
of which starch 10%, vegetables 40%

simple carbohydrates 0%

vegetable fat 10%

high in fibre

Salmon with broccoli, mangetout and wholewheat pasta

Fish provides the correct amount of protein in this meal, while the proportion of complex vegetable carbohydrates to complex starchy carbohydrates is balanced and the fibre content is substantial.

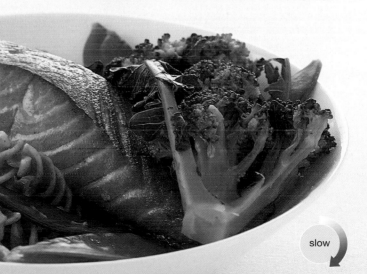

slow

glucose conversion

Complex versus simple carbohydrates

In the same way that there are two types of protein – complete and incomplete – there are also two types of carbohydrate. A complex carbohydrate is so-called because its fibre content remains intact. This means that its natural form has not been interfered with or changed in any way, or, if it has been processed at all, it is by a minimal amount. In contrast, a simple carbohydrate has been processed into a refined product and its fibre is lost. For example, if wheat grain is gently processed into wholemeal bread, it remains a complex carbohydrate. If the grain is polished further, it becomes a refined

product, white bread, which is classed as a simple carbohydrate. The same is true of brown rice and pasta compared to white rice and pasta, or an unsweetened muesli mix compared to a sugared, processed cereal.

When we think of carbohydrates we tend to think of starchy foods such as bread or potatoes, forgetting that fruits and vegetables are also carbohydrates. Complex vegetable carbohydrates are usually dense or green and leafy, such as broccoli and spinach. Some fruits, however, can be classed as simple carbohydrates if they have a low fibre content to start with. Since these fruits contain relatively little fibre to slow down the conversion rate to

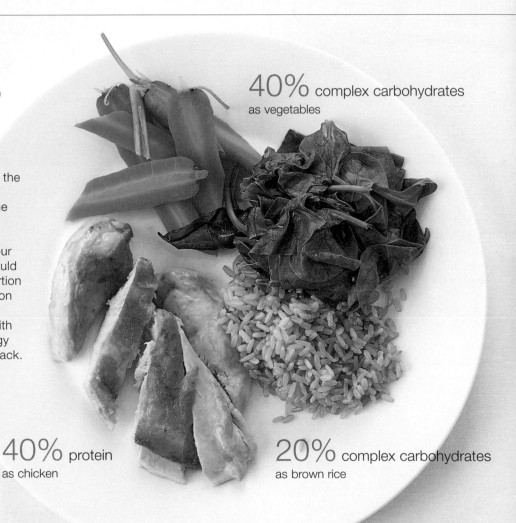

The correct proportions?

Lunch proportions

This lunchtime meal shows the ideal ratio of protein to complex carbohydrates. The size of chicken breast you should eat must be a little smaller than the palm of your hand, while vegetables should make up the largest proportion of complex carbohydrates on your plate. This balance of foods should supply you with enough nutrients and energy until your mid-afternoon snack.

40% complex carbohydrates as vegetables

40% protein as chicken

20% complex carbohydrates as brown rice

glucose, and are naturally high in sugar *(see pp.64–65),* they are broken down quickly inside the body. Examples of these fruits include watermelon and honeydew melon.

Correct ratios

By choosing the correct proportions of complete protein and complex carbohydrates, you can benefit from the energy generated by the slow release of glucose created from each meal or snack right up until it's time to eat again. And as complex carbohydrates contain plenty of fibre, each meal or snack helps to promote good digestive health, as well as energy and weight loss.

How do I get the proportions right?

Rather than having to weigh all your food, the portion of protein you should eat is a little smaller than the size of the palm of your hand. A piece of, say, chicken breast this size will supply 30–40 per cent of the total amount of food on your plate – the right protein requirement for an average person. However, we all require slightly differing amounts of protein and I have found that as much as 40–50 per cent protein works for me; you may thrive on less, or perhaps more. Complex carbohydrates complete the meal, although vegetables must, without fail, make up at least 60 per cent of these carbohydrates.

Dinner is different

There is just one exception to the rule about meal proportions. If you eat later on in the evening, I suggest that you avoid starchy carbohydrates altogether, since you won't use the energy they create. This means adding extra protein and vegetables to your evening meal so that the ratios are nearer to 50 per cent protein and 50 per cent vegetables.

I also recommend keeping a little portion of food back from your meal to snack on later – even if it's just a mouthful or two – to avoid those late night cravings with which you may be familiar.

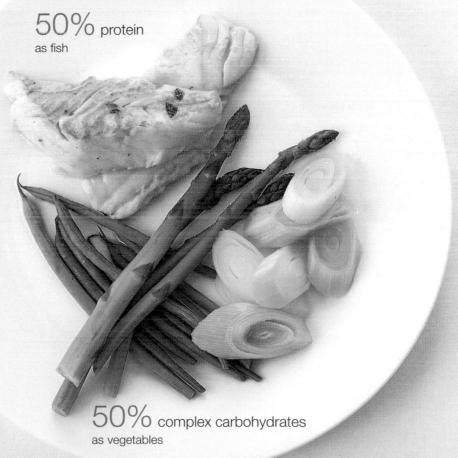

50% protein
as fish

50% complex carbohydrates
as vegetables

Protein profiles

The proteins that I recommend you should eat on the Plan for Life are all lean proteins, and are what is known as "complete". Remember that complete proteins cannot be generated by the body and must therefore come from your diet. The lean protein foods in the ideal category *(see chart, below)* contain all the essential amino acids.

Can I eat red meat?

I do not consider red meat to be a lean protein as it contains a higher proportion of saturated fats than, for example, skinless poultry. Saturated fats are not ideal for overall digestive health as they may promote the proliferation of unfriendly bacteria and yeasts in the intestines. However, red meat is classed as a complete protein and it is a good source of minerals, so eating red meat two or, if absolutely necessary, three times a week is a good way of maintaining some variety and interest in your choice of proteins.

Can I eat too much protein?

There is controversy as to whether you can eat too much protein, not least because diet plans based on 100 per cent protein plans do lead to weight loss – although the long-term cost to overall health is not yet fully understood. Too much protein can lead to a situation in which minerals are released from the bones to counteract the acidity of the blood. This is a natural occurrence when excess protein is eaten and can lead to reduced bone density. In addition, kidney damage is a risk for some individuals as the kidneys must cope with the added strain of breaking down large amounts of protein. Pure-protein diets are, by nature, low in fresh produce, so fibre and antioxidant intake is low as well.

A pure-protein diet is precisely the opposite of The Food Doctor plan, which has been designed to enhance digestive health and includes only about 40 per cent protein to meet most people's dietary requirements.

WHAT IS THE GLYCAEMIC INDEX?

The Glycaemic Index (GI) is, in effect, a list of the sugar content of foods. As a general rule, proteins and fats have low GI scores because the body takes longer to break them down into glucose. Carbohydrates have higher scores as they are broken down more rapidly.

Carbohydrates fall into two categories: simple and complex. Simple carbohydrates have had their fibre removed, while the fibre of complex carbohydrates remains intact. For example, apple juice is a simple carbohydrate because it is converted rapidly from food to glucose, but a whole apple remains a complex carbohydrate. The quicker the conversion, the higher the GI score *(see pp.52–53)*. So the juice has a high score and the fruit has a low score.

	MEAT & POULTRY	
Ideal choice These foods are all complete proteins and are therefore the best choice.	Duck eggs Hens' eggs Quails' eggs Calves' liver Lambs' liver Skinless chicken Skinless turkey Veal	
Good choice You can include these food choices frequently as part of a healthy diet.		
Adequate choice Eat these foods occasionally.	Bacon Beef Ham Lamb chops	Mince Pork chops

Why is fish so good for you?

Fish really does offer the best of both worlds. Not only is it an ideal source of protein, it is also rich in omega-3 essential fats. These fats have many functions in the body, but in terms of weight loss research has shown that such fats promote rather than hinder weight loss. Omega-3 fats also have an important role in promoting cardiovascular health, reducing the risk of Type 2 diabetes and enhancing brain function.

DAIRY	VEGETARIAN	FISH			
	Chick-peas	Anchovy	Gurnard	Marlin*	Sea bream
	Lentils	Bluefish*	Haddock	Monkfish	Skate
	Nuts (raw)	Bream	Hake	Orange roughy	Sprat*
	Quinoa	Brill	Halibut*	Perch*	Swordfish*
	Quorn	Carp*	Herring*	Plaice	Trout*
	Pumpkin seeds	Cod	Hoki	Red mullet*	Tuna*
	Sesame seeds	Dover sole	Lemon sole	Salmon*	Turbot
	Sunflower seeds	Eel*	Mackerel*	Sardine*	Whitebait*
	Tofu	Grey Mullet*	Mahi Mahi*	Sea bass	Whiting
Low-fat cottage cheese	Baked beans (unsweetened)				
Low-fat live natural yoghurt					
Full-fat yoghurt					
Hard cheese					

*Also a good source of omega-3 fats

Carbohydrate profiles

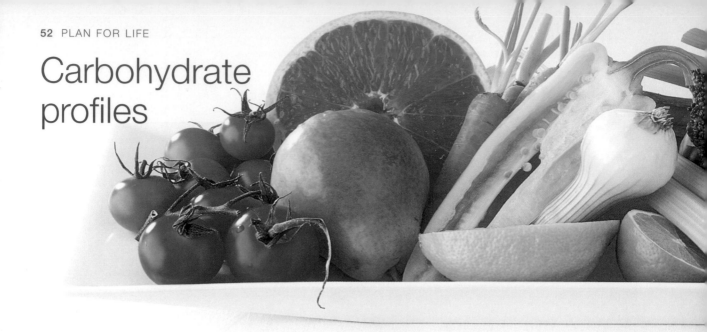

	GRAIN-BASED FOODS		FRUITS	
Ideal choice The complex carbohydrates at this level are ideal choices because they supply high levels of energy for longer *(see p.49)*. They are all broken down slowly into glucose by the body so they have a low GI score.	Barley Oatmeal Wholegrain rye bread		Apples Apricots (fresh) Blackberries Cranberries Grapefruit Lemons Limes	Pears Plums Strawberries
Good choice The foods in this category have a medium GI score and so they provide reasonably good levels of energy at a fairly steady rate.	Brown rice Couscous Granola bars containing nuts Pumpernickel bread Wholemeal bread Wholewheat pasta and spaghetti		Blueberries Cherries Grapes Loganberries Mangoes Oranges Papayas	Peaches Pineapples Tangerines
Adequate choice These carbohydrates are either refined, low in fibre, high in sugar or a combination of all three. As a result, they have a high GI score and provide only short-term energy.	Bagels Biscuits Breadsticks Breakfast cereals Croissants Doughnuts French bread Melba toast	Muffins White bread White pasta and spaghetti White rice	Bananas Dried fruit Figs Fruit juices Prunes	

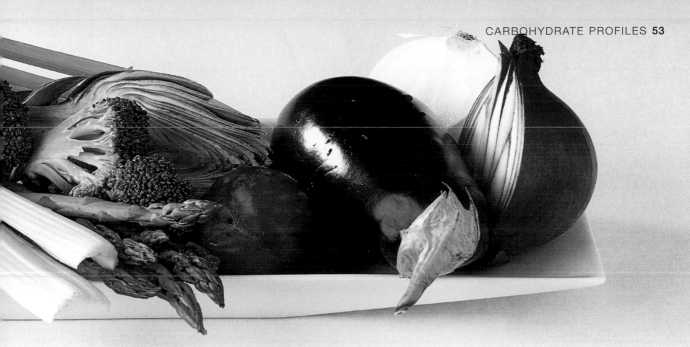

COOKED VEGETABLES		RAW FOODS	ALCOHOL
Artichokes	Leeks	Bean-sprouts	
Asparagus	Onions	Mushrooms	
Broccoli	Pak choi	Raw sprouted seeds and beans	
Brussels sprouts	Peppers	Tomatoes	
Cabbage	Spinach	Various salad leaves	
Cauliflower	String beans		
Greens			
Kale			
Carrots		Avocados	
Courgettes		Beetroot	
Kidney beans		Carrots	
Pumpkin		Celeriac	
Turnips		Olives	
Yellow squash			
Aubergines	Sweet potatoes		Beer
Parsnips	Yams		Spirits
Peas			Wine
Potatoes (baked, boiled, mashed)			
Squash			

Principle 2
Stay hydrated

We all know how important it is to drink plenty of water, and you should aim to drink at least six generously sized glasses or more of water a day. Water is also the best thirst-quencher; other beverages can only quench your thirst in proportion to the amount of water they contain.

There can be no doubt that keeping your fluid intake consistently high is imperative in order to aid weight loss. So does that mean drinking plain water only throughout the day? Many people ask me whether the water in tea, coffee, canned drinks, alcohol, juices and soups can count towards this fluid intake.

Regular tea and coffee contain caffeine, which has a mild diuretic effect and reduces overall hydration. So these drinks do not count towards your required fluid intake. Canned drinks, most of which are carbonated and probably sugared too, also don't count. Soups and juices do, but nothing beats water. Drink at least a litre and a half of water a day in addition to other liquids.

Limit your alcohol intake

Alcohol can have a detrimental effect on any weight-loss programme. Alcohol is a fermented product and as such can affect the levels of beneficial bacteria in the intestines *(see pp.8–11)*. It's also defined as a simple sugar, so it affects glucose levels quite rapidly – added to which it also acts as a dehydrating element.

The final blow is that alcohol reduces your resolve. In other words, even if you are following all ten principles and succeeding in your weight-loss plan, after a glass of alcohol your thoughts may wander to sugary, fatty foods, which can undermine all your good efforts. Having said that, alcohol is a part of life and can be an enjoyable social pastime, so there is a way to slot it into The Food Doctor plan. I suggest that you drink alcohol no more than three times a week and that you limit yourself to two glasses of wine or two measures of spirits without mixers, which are highly sugared. If you have been used

to drinking alcohol most days of the week, cutting down to a maximum of two or three times a week is an important first step. Wine is the best choice – although stay away from sweet wines – followed by pure vodka mixed with plenty of mineral water, ice and a squeeze of fresh lime juice (avoid lime cordial as this is also highly sugared). I do not recommend beers, stouts, lagers, or cider, all of which contain yeast, if not sugar, and can be detrimental to your overall digestive health.

Avoid salt

Excess salt intake can contribute to thirst, and the most likely sources of salt in the modern diet are ready-made meals. Since my weight-loss plan does not include such foods, your salt intake will automatically reduce. Stop adding salt in cooking or to your food, and use herbs (either dried or fresh), freshly ground black pepper or sugar-free mustards to flavour foods instead.

ALCOHOL: THE GOLDEN RULES

1 Never drink alcohol on an empty stomach. Drinking alcohol with food is preferable, so have your first drink when you start your meal to reduce the absorption of alcohol.

2 Drink alcohol no more than three times a week – preferably less.

3 Mix spirits with water and ice, not mixers or fruit juices.

4 Do not drink alcohol on two consecutive days.

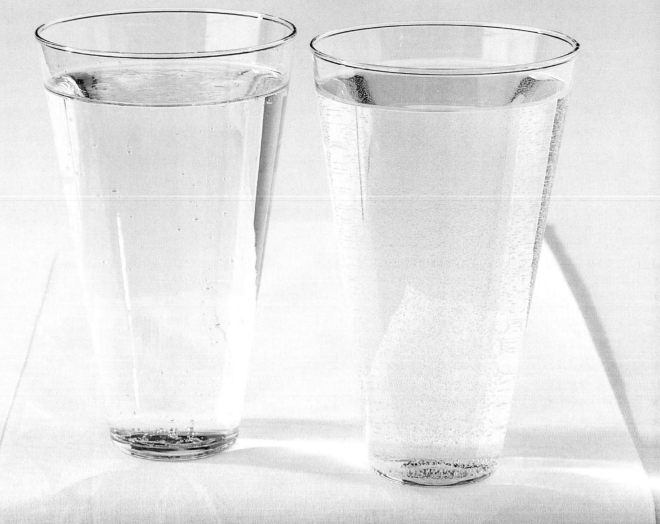

Tap or bottled water?

With regard to weight loss, there is little difference between choosing tap, bottled mineral or filtered water to drink as long as you ensure that you drink at least one litre of plain water a day in addition to juices and soups (totalling at least one and a half litres a day). This figure should be increased when you are exercising or during hot weather.

Still, rather than sparkling, water is my preferred choice of bottled mineral water as the gas contained in sparkling water can encourage bloating and discomfort in the gut.

Principle 3
Eat a wide variety of food

If you have a long-term weight issue, it's very possible that some foods have, over time, become off-limits in your mind, while you have grown to consider other foods "safe". This often tends to limit the range of foods you buy to just those that you feel most comfortable eating.

When I ask new clients to keep a food diary of their eating habits for a few days (see pp.16–17), all too often I am struck by the fact that they eat the same food nearly every day. In fact, for 90 per cent of the time most of us tend to buy the same small percentage – as little as 10 per cent – of foods available to us. We invariably shop, select and order food almost as if we are on autopilot, buying identical products week in, week out. Likewise, many weight-loss plans focus purely on a small group of foods. Perhaps in the past you have found that such dieting plans initially seem to work well when you eat the same food every day? Yet this strategy eventually makes any plan hard to follow, since you inevitably become bored and seek out foods from the so-called "forbidden list" that you know will satisfy you instead.

Why variety is important
It's vital that we eat a wide variety of foods in order to benefit from the wonderful array of nutrients that food offers. And in order to encourage a healthy relationship with food, I suggest that you be brave and try one new food every week. Some of the ideal foods listed in the proteins and carbohydrates charts (see pp.50–53) may be new to you, in which case I hope that you will try them. Similarly, although some of the ingredients listed in the recipe section (see pp.104–37) may not be familiar to you, please do try them.

So next time you are in the supermarket or at your local food market, buy something you have never tried before. You might want to flick through a recipe book first to look for something that appeals to you, or ask your shopkeeper how to cook what you have bought.

I am sure that once you begin to try a range of new foods you will enjoy eating many of them and add them regularly to your usual shopping list, thus making the meals you eat more varied and interesting.

The issue of grains
You may have noticed that grain-based foods do not feature heavily in the Seven-day Diet, and nor do they appear much in the long-term Plan for Life. The reason is that some grains contain elements that can easily aggravate the sensitive lining of the digestive tract.

FOOD INTOLERANCE
There is much discussion these days about how many wheat and dairy products people should eat. While I don't think that avoiding either food is altogether necessary for everyone, there is a strong case for becoming aware of just how much of one food you might be eating and whether it is causing inflammation in your intestines (see box, p.58). You may have a food intolerance if you suffer from any of the following symptoms:

- Bloating
- Irritable bowel syndrome (IBS)
- Dark circles under the eyes
- Excessive flatulence
- Runny nose
- Fatigue

Do you buy
the same food every week?

It's all too easy to become rooted in our shopping habits and repeatedly buy the same foods that we know and rely on. Ideally, however, we should all aim to eat one new food a week, be it a vegetable, fruit, grain, legume or herb. You may develop a taste for exciting new flavours and enjoy broadening your experience of foods.

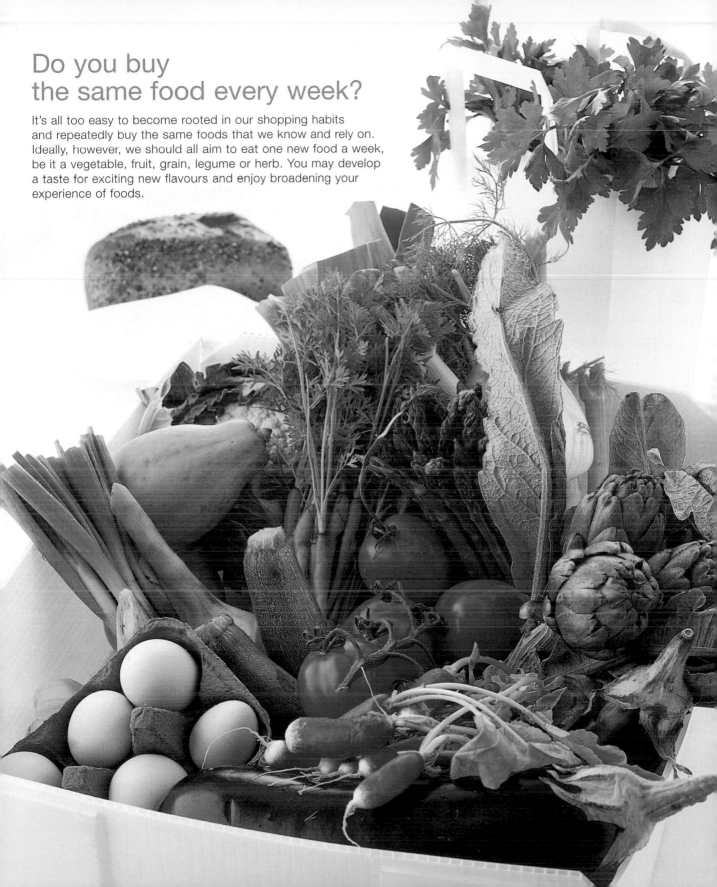

Gluten grains

Wheat, rye, barley and oats are known as gluten grains because they all contain "gliadin" in varying amounts. Gliadin is a substance found in gluten grains that can irritate the lining of the intestinal tract. Gluten is a sticky substance that helps to trap the air in bread, ensuring that it expands and has the correct feel. In recent years, grains have been cross-bred to produce new variants with a higher gluten content. If you look at the grain family tree *(see below),* you will notice that wheat, barley, oats and rye are closely related, and rice slightly less so, while corn, millet and cane sugar are from the other side of the family.

Over the years, I have worked with many clients who have benefited enormously from minimizing their intake of grains, especially those containing gluten. Having said that, grains are included in small amounts in both the Seven-day Diet and the Plan for Life because they are good sources of fibre and are rich in B vitamins, both of which aid weight loss. So do eat some wheat products, but keep the amounts as low as you can. Where possible, try to vary your grains. For example, buy 100 per cent rye bread one week, yeast-free soda bread the next and wholegrain brown bread the week after that.

White pasta, made from refined wheat, is often served and eaten in large quantities. If you want to eat pasta, have a few strands as part of a meal – much as you would have some potatoes or a spoonful of rice. Avoid eating a whole bowl of pasta, even if it's just as a starter. When you shop, buy wholewheat pasta, which is a complex carbohydrate, or try products made from corn or rice flour (a word of warning: they do not have the same consistency as wheat pasta and are more likely to be soft than *al dente*).

WHEAT AND WEIGHT PROBLEMS

There does seem to be a link between wheat intake and weight problems for some people. Wheat contains around 45 per cent gliadin, the substance that can cause irritation and lead to mild inflammation of the lining of the gut. If you think that wheat may be linked to any digestive problems you have, visit an appropriate nutrition professional for advice. Even if you do not have a food intolerance, vary your intake of grains weekly.

THE RELATIONSHIP OF MAJOR CEREAL GRAINS

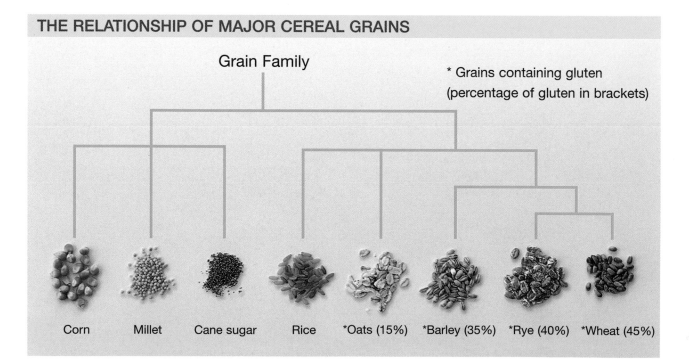

Grain Family

* Grains containing gluten
(percentage of gluten in brackets)

Corn   Millet   Cane sugar   Rice   *Oats (15%)   *Barley (35%)   *Rye (40%)   *Wheat (45%)

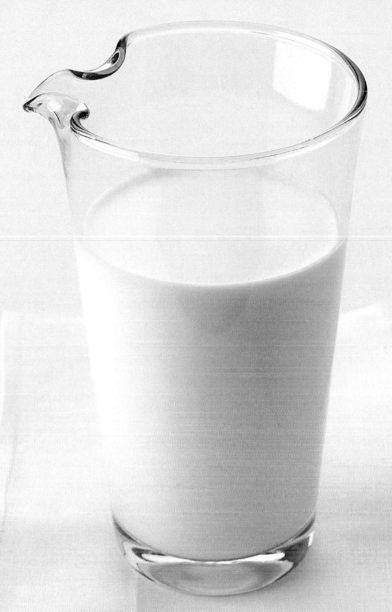

How much dairy should I have?

Many diets exclude dairy products but, as my aim is to encourage you to eat a wide variety of foods, I suggest that you include dairy products from time to time. If you are concerned about the possibility of food intolerance from dairy products, you need to vary the dairy products you eat at home, so that day to day you don't have too much of, say, cows' milk. If you follow this advice, you needn't be worried about avoiding dishes with cows' milk when you dine out.

Principle 4
Fuel up frequently

You are probably becoming used to the idea that if you eat the right amount of food combinations that are broken down into glucose slowly, you will create a consistent supply of energy and still be able to lose weight. But it's not just the foods and amounts that are important, it's the timing too.

Eating little and often is a crucial element of my plan. By eating the right foods and snacks at regular intervals through the day, you should be able to keep your energy levels constant so that you can function well without food cravings – the downfall of so many dieters.

The benefits explained

In the same way that you need to eat proteins with complex carbohydrates to maximize the benefits of a healthy diet and minimize the frequency of insulin production (see p.12), so fuelling up frequently ensures

ENERGY TIMELINE

The pink line on this energy timeline depicts the range of highs and lows that a typical person will experience through the day. Set against those peaks and troughs is the stabilizing green line of The Food Doctor plan, which illustrates how eating the right foods at certain times can help you avoid the lows that might otherwise occur, and keep your energy levels constant.

THE FOOD DOCTOR PLAN

AVERAGE DIET

This breakfast of natural yoghurt, seeds and pear tops up your energy levels after a night's sleep.

A snack of cold vegetable omelette left over from last night's supper keeps you going through the morning.

Processed cereal for breakfast sends your blood-glucose levels soaring, then soon leaves you hungry again.

A piece of fruit such as a watermelon is high in sugar and low in fibre, and so makes an insubstantial snack.

| 08:00 | 09:00 | 10:00 | 11:00 | 12:00 |

that a steady supply of glucose enters the bloodstream to be converted into energy. Together, these two factors create a potent mix of the right food at the right time, leading to effective weight loss and stable energy levels.

How it works in practice

Within two hours of eating breakfast your blood-glucose levels begin to drop. These levels continue to diminish until they reach a low point that the body interprets as hunger. There is an optimal period of time just before you begin to feel the pangs of hunger, and it is during this time that eating something satisfying and healthy will make all the difference to your energy levels. This may mean that you have to teach yourself to recognize the first signs of hunger, which can take a number of forms ranging from loss of concentration to feeling slightly shaky. If you have dieted previously, you will be familiar with the big mid-morning dip depicted in the diagram below. If, however, you follow The Food Doctor plan and choose to eat an appropriate snack *(see pp.82–83)* mid way through the morning, you will be able to combat a slight dip in energy levels and any associated symptoms of hunger.

Ideally, you should eat approximately every two or three hours through the day. So you need to eat a proper lunch and another healthy snack in the middle of the afternoon before your evening meal.

Think of this principle as the equivalent of filling up your car with just enough premium grade fuel to last you to the next filling station, and then doing the same again and again throughout the day. In this way you can combat hunger pangs and bad food choices, minimize insulin production, maximize your energy levels and lose weight, all at the same time.

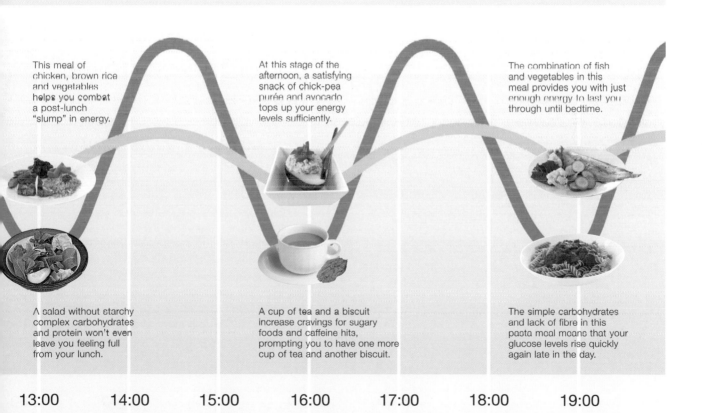

This meal of chicken, brown rice and vegetables helps you combat a post-lunch "slump" in energy.

At this stage of the afternoon, a satisfying snack of chick-pea purée and avocado tops up your energy levels sufficiently.

The combination of fish and vegetables in this meal provides you with just enough energy to last you through until bedtime.

A salad without starchy complex carbohydrates and protein won't even leave you feeling full from your lunch.

A cup of tea and a biscuit increase cravings for sugary foods and caffeine hits, prompting you to have one more cup of tea and another biscuit.

The simple carbohydrates and lack of fibre in this pasta meal means that your glucose levels rise quickly again late in the day.

13:00   14:00   15:00   16:00   17:00   18:00   19:00

Principle 5
Eat breakfast

Unlike many diets that leave you hungry and craving forbidden foods, this diet plan promotes eating little and often as the key to keeping your energy levels consistent and achieving successful weight loss. So it is essential that at the start of each day you eat a healthy breakfast.

Skipping any meal is one step to failure, and by far the worst meal to skip is breakfast. You may not have much of an appetite first thing and I appreciate that mornings can be stressful with kids to organize as well as getting yourself ready for work, but investing time in eating breakfast is fundamental to losing weight.

Time for a change
If you are the sort of person who has a cup of tea or coffee and a bowl of processed breakfast cereal to kick-start your day, then the time has come to make some changes to your diet.

Let's look at what this typical breakfast does to your body. The cereal almost certainly lacks protein. It is converted into glucose rapidly by the body, and so produces only short-term energy. Coupled with the caffeine, it may make you feel satisfied, but only for a short time. If you eat breakfast at 8am, by 10am it is likely that you will experience an energy slump, which is perceived as hunger. If you have another cup of coffee and a biscuit or two, the whole cycle starts again. As the Plan for Life is designed to help you feel energetic and reduce hunger pangs, your intake of caffeinated drinks and sugary foods should be kept to a minimum.

A better approach
Eating the right foods little and often is the key to increased energy and sustained weight loss. If you eat a healthy breakfast, such as muesli or natural yoghurt with fruit and seeds, you shouldn't feel hungry until 10.30–11am, which is the best time to eat a snack in order to sustain your energy levels. These types of breakfasts are easy to prepare and have the right combination of food groups: the nuts, seeds and yoghurt provide your body with plenty of protein and the wholegrains are rich in complex carbohydrates. If you do not enjoy yoghurt or muesli, there are many other healthy options for breakfast, including eggs, toast, crackers, fruit and smoothies. See pages 78–79 for a range of suggestions to inspire you. Whatever you decide to eat, remember that taking a few minutes to eat a good breakfast is essential and sets the scene for the rest of the day.

CAN I HAVE COFFEE?

I love coffee and I feel that no morning is complete without it. As long as you have coffee with or after a meal or snack containing protein and fibre, you should be able to keep your energy levels high. However, do not have more than one or two cups a day because caffeine stimulates your adrenal glands to produce adrenaline. This is the same response your body has under stress, and is part of what is known as the "flight or fight" response – providing short-term energy, a heightened sense of sight and hearing and quickened responses. Once the "danger" has passed, adrenaline production stops, energy levels drop and you may experience fatigue and hunger, which in turn encourages you to make poor food choices. Try to limit yourself to one cup a day, and don't add sugar to your drink. By now your sugar cravings should be manageable, so it shouldn't be too hard.

Is your breakfast balanced?

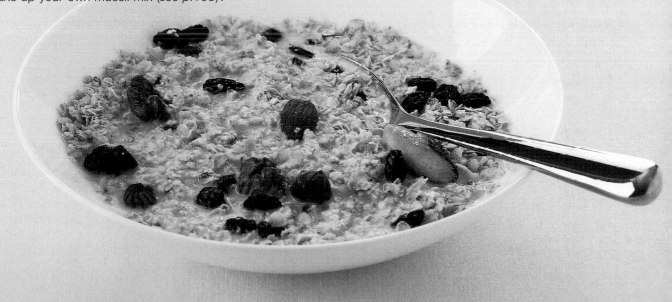

My preferred choice of milk

I suggest that you buy whole milk for your breakfasts and drinks instead of semi-skimmed and skimmed milk. I find whole milk more satisfying than skimmed milk, especially when you consider that there isn't much difference between the two in terms of fat content.

The ideal muesli

Choose a muesli that contains plenty of nuts and seeds and not too much dried fruit, since this combination will be broken down into glucose relatively slowly. Or, rather than buying ready-made muesli, why not visit your local health-food store and buy the ingredients separately to make up your own muesli mix (see p.108)?

Principle 6
Avoid sugar

I believe that sugar is just as much to blame for weight gain as is fat. You will benefit enormously by cutting down on the amount of sugar in your diet and, as The Food Doctor plan is designed to help you achieve good digestive health, avoiding sugar takes on added importance.

It is worth explaining exactly what I mean by the word "sugar". There are many variations on the white or brown granules that you buy in packets, such as sorbitol, malt and even honey *(see box, below)*. With so many different names for sugar, it's no wonder that most people have little idea just how much of it may be present in their diet.

The aim of limiting your sugar intake is to reduce the amount and frequency of insulin secretion in the body. Sugar in all its forms is broken down by the digestive system into glucose extremely quickly. As the blood-glucose levels suddenly rise high in response, they trigger the production of insulin *(see p.12),* which in turn forces the glucose levels down again by converting the glucose into fat through a series of biochemical changes. This is the reason why we need to minimize insulin production if we want to lose weight. Foods that are converted into glucose rapidly should be avoided or, at the very least, combined with those that are broken down at a slower rate.

The fat-free myth
Sugars of one kind or another are almost always added to processed and ready-made foods, and it's not uncommon for a product to contain several different types of sugar. The more sugar there is in a product, the less fat it contains, which allows manufacturers to claim that it is low in fat or that it contains less than a certain percentage of fat. In reality, this means that in your desire to lose weight you buy, for example, a product that is labelled 95 per cent fat-free. You have probably done so for years. So why don't you become the thin person you want to be when all you eat is this type of food? The answer is that the sugars in these products are always higher when the fat content has been decreased.

How the theory works
Let's see how this theory works in practice. You choose a low-fat muffin for breakfast or a snack *(see right)*. As its sugar content is higher than that of a regular muffin your blood-glucose levels rise sharply and fall quickly, leaving you hungry again all too soon. You battle with your food cravings, give in and eat another low-fat snack.

If you eat a meal or snack containing complete protein and complex carbohydrates *(see pp.46–53),* the insulin produced is minimal by comparison. Your prolonged energy levels and reduced hunger pangs even enable you to make sensible choices about what to eat next.

ALTERNATIVE NAMES FOR SUGAR

Although these substances are derived from a variety of sources, they are all classed as sugars.

- Sucrose
- Mannitol
- Glucose
- Honey
- Lactose
- Fructose
- Sorbitol
- Corn syrup
- Malt
- Malt extract
- Maltose
- Rice syrup
- Rice extract
- Molasses
- Golden syrup
- Invert sugar

Can I use artificial sweeteners instead?

Sweeteners are usually added to so-called diet drinks and processed foods. In The Food Doctor plan you won't be eating any of these foods, so the issue of sweeteners shouldn't come up. If you add sweeteners to your tea and coffee, I suggest that you try to stop. Sweeteners have no nutritional value and can affect the overall benefits of the Plan for Life by perpetuating any cravings you might have for sweet foods.

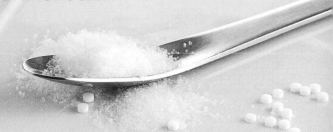

Which is the best option?

If you choose to eat a low-fat muffin, its calorie count may be low but check its sugar content against a regular muffin. The low-fat muffin almost certainly contains a higher percentage of sugars, and thus it is classed as a simple carbohydrate. The body can convert it from food to glucose with ease. As a result, blood-glucose levels rise and insulin is released, which in turn increases fat stores in the body.

Full-fat cranberry muffin

A full-fat muffin is typically made of white flour, sugar and fat. Any fruit, such as cranberries, or fibre, such as bran, supplies a small amount of complex carbohydrates.

simple carbohydrates 80%
of which sugar 40%, white flour 40%

vegetable fat 15%

complex carbohydrates 5%

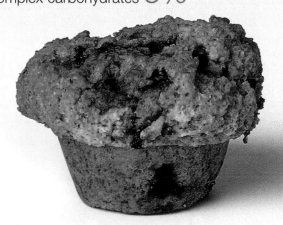

Low-fat cranberry muffin

This low-fat muffin may now contain less saturated fat, but to compensate far more sugar has been added during the manufacturing process.

simple carbohydrates 90%
of which sugar 60%, white flour 40%

vegetable fat 5%

complex carbohydrates 5%

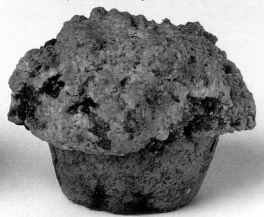

Principle 7
Exercise is essential

A weight-loss programme will not prove to be very successful if you don't exercise, just as exercising frequently while eating the wrong foods isn't likely to result in a healthier lifestyle either. Even with the busiest schedule there is time to do more if you want to, so make exercise a priority.

My expertise is in food, not in exercise, but I do know that the benefits of exercising are far-reaching, and not just in the area of weight-loss. A regular exercise programme can help reduce the risk of cardiovascular disease, osteoporosis and Type 2 diabetes. Exercise can even help you cope with stress more effectively.

Adjusting your metabolic rate
Exercise increases your metabolic rate, that is, the speed at which your body uses up food as energy. Likewise, the aim of exercise in the context of The Food Doctor plan is to increase the rate at which the food you eat, and any stores of fat, are utilized for energy.

Remember that this eating plan relies on supplying premium-grade fuel in the form of whole foods to the body, where it is converted into glucose and circulated in the bloodstream to cells to be used as fuel for energy production. On my Plan for Life, the rate of glucose entering the cells is steady enough to keep energy levels consistent and avoid lows (which we interpret as hunger).

However, it is possible to influence how that glucose, or fuel, is managed at cellular level. In each cell there is a tiny power plant, called a mitochondria, which effectively converts the glucose into energy. Cells are amazingly advanced structures that respond to requirement, so if you increase your energy output, the cells respond accordingly by creating more of these tiny mitochondria in each cell to make yet more energy. Thus you can affect how much glucose is used up as energy. Exercising encourages this smooth conversion of glucose into energy because consistent and increased energy helps your body burn off that unwanted fat.

What sort of exercise is best?
I am a firm believer that you should always consult an appropriate professional if you need advice about what sort of exercise to undertake. I wouldn't suggest taking nutritional advice from instructors else unless they are fully qualified, and since I am not an expert in exercise I only make suggestions as to what might suit you.

If you decide to join a gym, ask a trained instructor to help you devise a simple routine that you can stick to and enjoy, since I have found that, even with the best intentions, the gym can sometimes become boring after a while. Try to vary your exercise routine, or exercise with a friend who has similar goals to your own. This makes it more fun, and you can chat as you exercise.

Depending on your current level of fitness, you could also try jogging, aerobic classes, swimming, walking the dog or playing football, tennis or squash. The list is endless.

If the thought of exercising is abhorrent to you, then start off gently. Try walking to your local shops every other day instead of taking the car, or getting off the bus or train a stop early on the way to work and walking briskly the rest of the way. As long as you exercise for a minimum of 30 minutes, three times a week, the exercise you choose isn't that important. You needn't punish yourself in the gym. Instead you must raise your heartbeat to a level at which you break out in a sweat at some point over the half hour, but while still being able to continue a conversation.

So, be creative with your choice of exercise because the benefits are many and because your progress with The Food Doctor plan will be greatly enhanced.

What to eat after exercise?

You may well find that you feel hungrier if you are exercising regularly. I suggest that you increase your portion sizes a little at mealtimes to match this, but by no more than ten per cent. You should also ensure that you have appropriate snacks to eat immediately after you have exercised: it is especially important to replenish spent glucose levels after any exercise, so eat something that contains complex carbohydrates as well as protein, such as a cereal bar that contains oats, fruit, nuts and seeds.

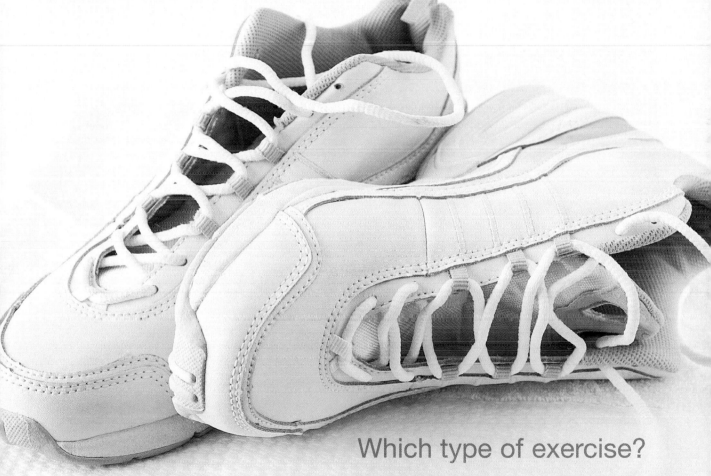

Which type of exercise?

The bottom line is that you must be physically active, be it swimming, jogging, playing tennis, football, squash, going to the gym or simply walking. You should aim to complete at least 30 minutes of any form of exercise three times a week or more. This will help to raise your metabolic rate and improve your overall digestion, helping you to get rid of any fat stores that you have accumulated.

Principle 8
Follow the 80:20 rule

Perhaps you have followed diets in the past that revolve around sticking to the prescribed plan 100 per cent of the time. The problem is that it's in our nature to veer off course after a while – usually out of frustration or boredom – hence the all-important 80:20 rule.

The Food Doctor plan encourages you to eat little and often so that your hunger pangs are minimized and you are unlikely to suffer from food cravings.

However, life just isn't that easy, as we all know, and from time to time you will eat out of line with the plan. I know that however many practical suggestions for coping with special occasions, interesting recipes or sound advice this book contains, there will be times when nothing will work for you apart from your chosen treat, be it chocolate cake, sweets or ice cream. The good news is that this is entirely possible, within reason.

Putting the rule into practice

So what constitutes the 80:20 rule? If you follow the Plan for Life principles – such as combining the right food groups and avoiding refined carbohydrates and sugars – as closely as possible, then I believe that your food will satisfy you and your success rate will be high. By eating regularly to keep blood-glucose levels more even, you won't want to eat the sort of foods you probably see as treats now. Yet the experience of eating goes further than just supplying energy. Follow the plan for 80 per cent of the time and you will still achieve success, albeit more slowly. For example, if you eat healthily through the day, you can save your remaining 20 per cent for when you are out to dinner or at a party. There is more information about this in special situations (*see pp.92–95*).

Try not to veer from The Food Doctor plan every day as this could create a habit in which you crave the wrong types of food. As a consequence, eating in line with the Plan for Life will become harder to do and the possibility of slipping back into old habits increases. On average, use the 80:20 rule to treat yourself two or three times a week, perhaps taking into account any situations you may have coming up that mean you can't eat what you would ideally like.

EATING OUT

When you have a choice about where to eat, stick to a restaurant or café that you know will enable you to eat in line with the Plan for Life principles. It's possible to eat well nearly everywhere as long as you keep food proportions in your mind when ordering. For example, have a vegetable-based starter without pastry and a complete protein for your main course. If you have no choice as to the venue, then hopefully you can allocate your 20 per cent quota to this meal. If not, then eat as carefully as you can and make up for it later.

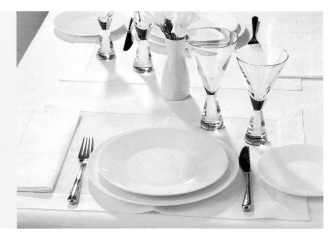

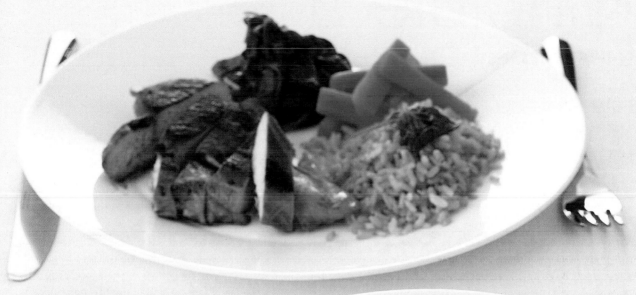

What can I do about chocolate?

Chocolate tends to be by far the one food that is craved more than any other, and it can be the downfall of so many dieters. Here are some guidelines to follow.

- The pleasure in eating chocolate should come from the flavour of the bean, not from the fats and sugar that make up around 80 per cent of many popular brands.

- If you crave chocolate, eat a couple of squares of the richest, darkest variety you can find – preferably one that contains more than 70 per cent cocoa. The higher the bean content, the lower the sugar and fat content. Two squares of dark chocolate are far more satisfying than lesser varieties.

- If you are the sort of person who can't eat just two squares of chocolate, try buying mini bars or breaking off two chunks and putting the rest out of sight and reach.

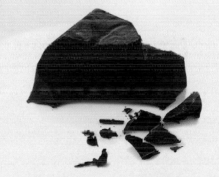

Principle 9
Make time to eat

Eating is an essential yet pleasurable social ritual, and one that I feel has become devalued in our society. Fast food, ready-made meals and the pressure we all impose on ourselves to save time have eliminated the importance of sitting down to enjoy a meal. So make time to eat.

I have had consultations with many clients who, while they are accountable in other areas of their lives as parents or employees, for example, seem to take no interest in or responsibility for what they eat. Ironically, some of these clients will change their eating habits if they find that they are pregnant, or planning pregnancy, only to change back again after their baby is born. This is often in spite of feeling much better on the healthier eating plan while pregnant.

I have also worked with many families who rush through dinner, both cooking and eating their meal, simply so that they can spend the rest of the evening in front of the television watching cookery programmes!

Modern life appears to have taken the pleasure out of cooking and eating food. It seems to be something that is not worth fussing over and it wastes valuable time: let the food manufacturers do your work for you so that you can do something else more important instead. If this lifestyle sounds familiar to you, then ask yourself how ready-made meals and processed foods have contributed to your weight problems. If you learn to value and respect good food, making time to eat will become normal practice for you and your family. Try to sit down and eat at least one meal a day together. Take your time eating, and you may even find that you linger at the table chatting after your meal is over.

Eating at work

If your job is stressful and you never get a chance to eat a proper meal, you will probably snack when you can and rush through a sandwich at lunchtime. However, on The Food Doctor plan I want you to eat little and often, and this means eating mid-morning and mid-afternoon snacks that may require you to leave your desk and take a few minutes to prepare and eat them (see pp.82–83). You may need to plan ahead in the early stages until you become used to the plan, but your snack doesn't have to be complicated or take more than a minute to prepare. More importantly, taking the time to eat properly and chew well will ensure that you supply yourself with enough energy to see you through until your next meal.

If you really cannot leave your desk, keep a bag of raw, unsalted nuts in your drawer and measure a palmful of them in your hand to eat with an apple. If you have appointments or meetings throughout the day, try to leave a gap of a few minutes between them so that you can eat. If you don't, you are more likely to rely on coffee and biscuits and then make a poor food choice at lunchtime because your energy levels will be low and need to be replenished quickly.

THE BENEFITS OF TAKING TIME TO EAT

- Your stress levels are reduced.

- Chewing slowly and thoroughly enables you to digest your food properly and maintain good digestive health.

- Your body can absorb the nutrients from your food more effectively.

- A feeling of satisfaction that you have eaten a tasty, filling meal.

Why should I stop to eat at work?

Try to view eating your lunch or snack at work as a separate activity that you should concentrate on – don't treat it as an adjunct or an afterthought. You must take the time to eat slowly and digest your food properly, so stop working or close down your computer while you eat.

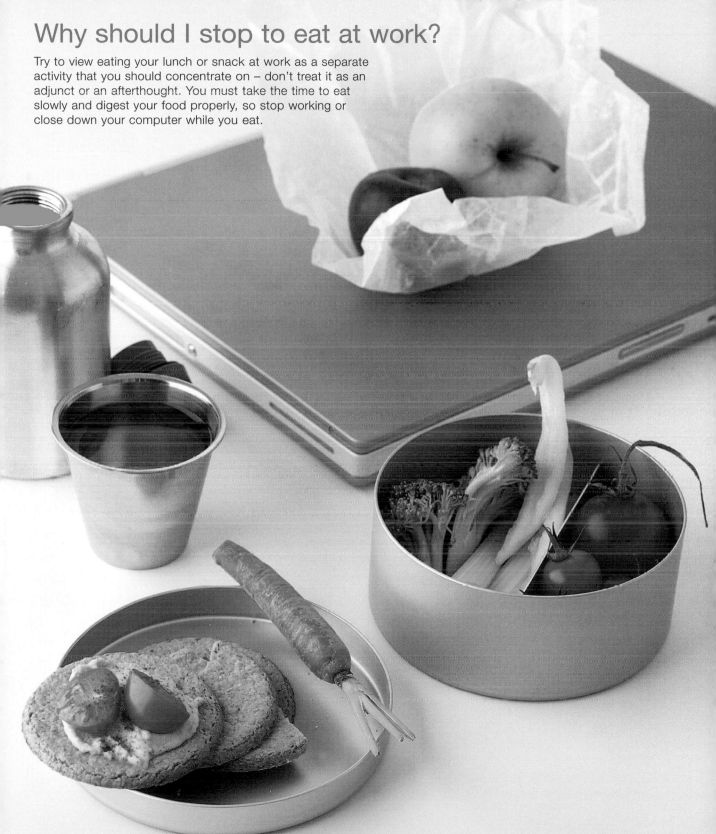

Principle 10
Eat fat to lose fat

If you come from a background of calorie-counting, you probably see fat as the enemy. Yet although the fat accumulated in our bodies and the fats in food are, in theory, similar, they are actually quite different: the essential fats present in a variety of foods are crucial for the body to function properly.

Fat contains nine calories per gram, the highest calorie count of any food there is, and this is why many diet plans advocate limiting your intake of fatty foods. However, I believe that it is saturated fats, not the all-important essential fats, that should be avoided.

What's the difference?

There are many types of fats that the body uses in a variety of different ways. Some fats are termed "essential" as they must come from the food we eat *(see right)*. The conversion of these essential fats into substances that can be used internally is dependent upon several enzymes, which themselves require specific nutrients in order to work efficiently. Even those fats that are deemed non-essential to the body have a role to play, although saturated fats are not required in any great amount. Furthermore, fat adds to the satisfaction of eating –

known in the food industry as "mouth feel" – and is considered a vital part of the eating experience. When we eat fat a substance called galanin, which actually increases our desire to eat more fat, is released into the body. This is why we often crave fatty foods, and why they are so pleasurable to eat. Luckily, this same feeling is experienced when we eat essential fats, which should form the bulk of our fat intake.

How much is too much?

Research has shown that a diet supplying not more than 30 per cent of energy from fat is the best way to lose weight. So you will find that by including 20 per cent of fat in the form of essential fats in your diet you will still enjoy the satisfaction of eating, yet the rate at which your food is converted into glucose is slowed down, thus fitting in perfectly with the Plan for Life principles.

LOW-FAT FOOD LABELS

If you buy, for example, a packet of crisps that claims to be low in fat, you may see something like "33 per cent less fat" advertised on the packet. The food label (*see top right*) lists the product as containing just over five grams of fat, but this figure does not take into account the number of calories you will eat. Bear in mind that fat contains nine calories per gram, and the total calorie count of this product is 113 calories. When you eat the crisps, you must multiply five grams by

Per 24g bag	
Energy	113 calories
Protein	1.8 g
Carbohydrates	14.4 g
of which sugars	0.1g
Fats	5.3g

Per 24g bag	
Energy	113 calories
Fats	45 calories
Calories from fat	42%

nine calories to determine how much energy this food supplies – in this case it is 45 calories. That's how many calories are provided by fat alone in this product, which is what the label should really say (*see bottom left*). So although the fat, by weight, is about three grams less than a regular bag of crisps, the percentage of calories from fat is still high: 42 per cent of the total calorie count. You are only eating five grams of fat by weight, but 42 per cent of all the calories in the product comes from fat.

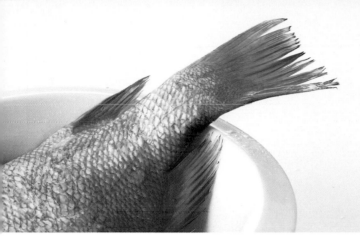

Which fats are good?

Foods that contain essential fats

Overall, the fats that are naturally found in fish (such as salmon, mackerel, tuna, trout, eel and sardines), raw nuts, seeds and olives are those that are most beneficial to your diet. However, don't go overboard with these foods: keep an eye on how much you are eating, and aim to eat no more than a palmful of nuts daily and fish four or five times a week.

The good oils

All of the foods illustrated below are good sources of valuable essential fats In thelr most natural form. In addition, the oils derived from these foods are beneficial in small quantities. Choose cold-pressed, good-quality oils as the basis for salad dressings and marinades, and avoid cooking with these oils at high temperatures as this causes them to lose their nutritional value.

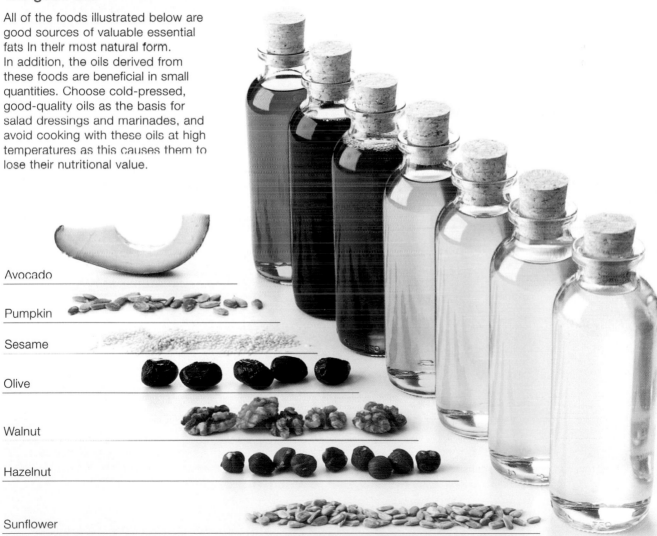

Avocado

Pumpkin

Sesame

Olive

Walnut

Hazelnut

Sunflower

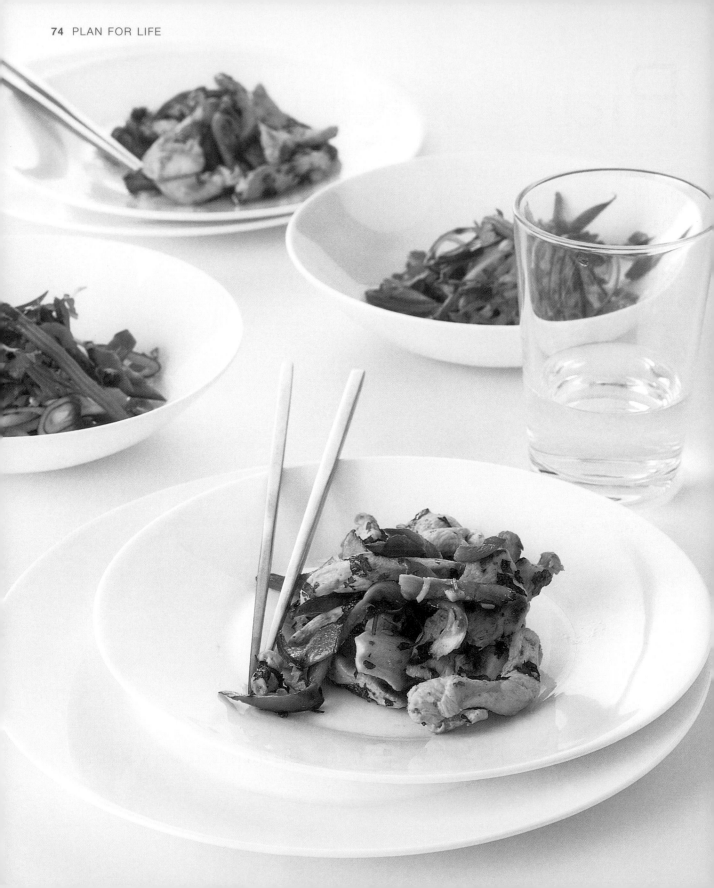

Planning meals

This part of the book explains the practice behind the theory of the Plan for Life. The information in this section reminds you of the main aims for each mealtime – what you should be eating, and when – in order to sustain your energy levels and maintain a healthy digestive system. To help you remember the food groups in The Food Doctor plan, which consist of complete proteins, starchy complex carbohydrates and complex carbohydrates in the form of vegetables, look at my food equations. These equations will help you to think carefully about which categories your food choices fall into, and whether they are really healthy enough to be part of this eating plan.

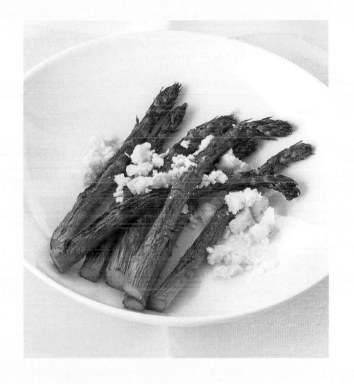

Deciding what to eat

The selections of suggested meal and snack options will hopefully provide a springboard to encourage you to think for yourself when deciding what you should eat each mealtime. These suggestions combine the food groups in the ratios that I feel are ideal for maximizing energy, reducing hunger and promoting weight loss. Feel free to substitute any protein for another according to your preference, and always include vegetables at lunch and dinner and with snacks to ensure that you don't end up on a very high-protein diet.

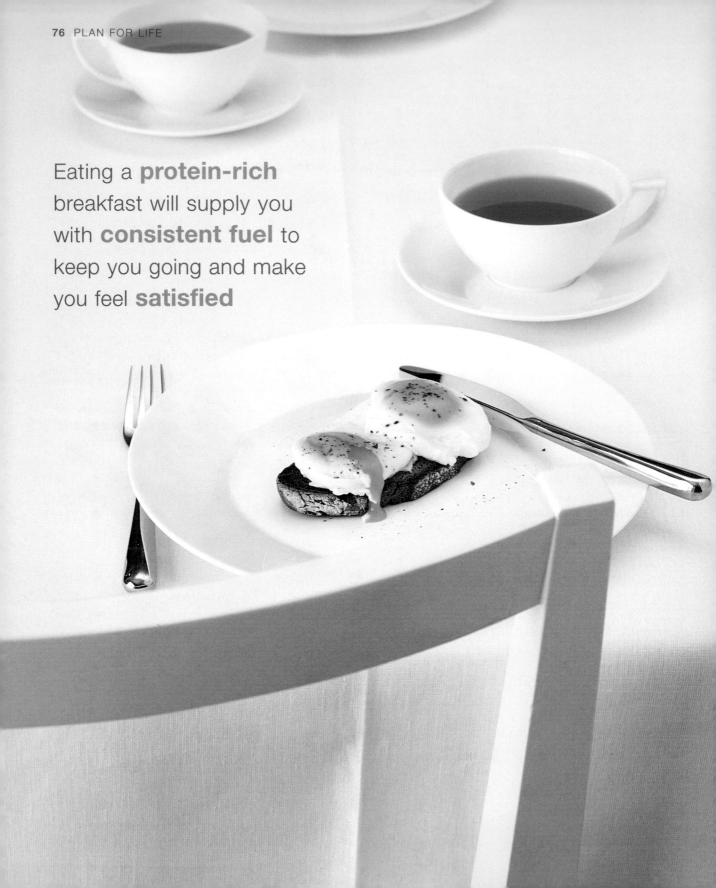

Eating a **protein-rich** breakfast will supply you with **consistent fuel** to keep you going and make you feel **satisfied**

Breakfast

We have already examined the principle of eating breakfast and how it sets the scene for rest of the day *(see pp.62–63)*, but let's look more closely at how this theory works and why it is such a fundamental and important principle to establish.

The food you eat is broken down by your digestive system into its component parts – glucose, vitamins, minerals, and so on. It is glucose that creates energy and acts as the fuel for every cell, so the breakfast you eat is responsible for providing you with energy for a significant part of the morning. In order to lose weight you must eat the right ratio of food groups *(see p.48)* to ensure that glucose is released gradually into the bloodstream. This steady release limits the production of insulin, which must be minimized if body fat is to be reduced accordingly.

What is a healthy breakfast?

Having established that breakfast must include some foods that are broken down slowly by the body, the reality is that conventional breakfast foods usually comprise caffeine and simple carbohydrates, which supply a quick energy surge and little more. The image of a "healthy" breakfast of cereal, toast, orange juice and black coffee is, in fact, based on the theory of calorie counting, and does not include any protein. I can almost guarantee that this type of breakfast will not meet your energy requirements for the morning: as the

glucose created from this food runs out, your body interprets this signal as hunger and you begin an eating cycle of desire and denial.

Eating a protein-rich breakfast will supply you with consistent fuel to keep you feeling satisfied so that you don't become overly hungry. Remember that this is a protein-rich breakfast, not a pure protein one, so include some complex carbohydrates too. This sort of meal isn't always as instant as a packet of cereal, so turn to pages 78–79 for some ideas and then put aside a few extra minutes each day to make a proper breakfast.

THE FOOD DOCTOR BREAKFAST EQUATION

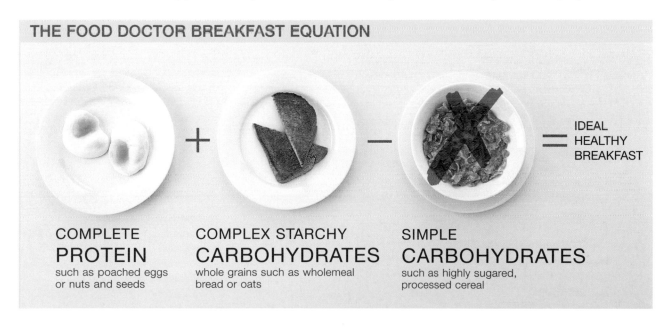

COMPLETE PROTEIN
such as poached eggs or nuts and seeds

+

COMPLEX STARCHY CARBOHYDRATES
whole grains such as wholemeal bread or oats

−

SIMPLE CARBOHYDRATES
such as highly sugared, processed cereal

=

IDEAL HEALTHY BREAKFAST

Breakfast suggestions

Many of us tend to view breakfast as a time-consuming event that keeps us from starting the day, but it is important to remember that this meal is vital if you want to maintain high energy levels through the morning. These suggestions are easy to prepare, yet are satisfying and taste good.

By now you should be familiar with the principle that protein combined with complex carbohydrates will provide a healthy, energy-giving meal (*see pp.46–49*). This is a crucial requirement for the first meal of the day. For example, if you have a piece of fish left over from your supper the night before and you want to eat it for your breakfast, there is nothing to say that you shouldn't have it. It's not a typical choice, perhaps, but it fits in with The Food Doctor plan. You must eat some complex carbohydrates with the fish, so you could either have a mouthful or two of vegetables, a couple of rice crackers or a piece of rye toast. Here are some simple suggestions which may inspire you.

Hot breakfasts

Two eggs scrambled, poached or soft-boiled with a slice of rye toast or rice crackers
Eggs supply the protein in this meal, while the toast or crackers provide the complex carbohydrates. Alternatively, you might like to try poached eggs with grilled tomatoes and mushrooms. If you don't have time to cook in the morning, hard-boil some eggs the night before and leave them to cool. At breakfast time chop up the eggs, add chopped fresh herbs such as dill or tarragon and eat them with a piece of toast or two oatcakes.

Porridge
A sustaining meal of porridge will provide you with some of the necessary fibre required for a healthy digestive system. Add protein in the form of a tablespoon of live natural yoghurt and mix in some chopped pear to provide more complex carbohydrates (this also gives it added taste) – or try an easy recipe for hot apple oats (*see p.106*).

Fish with grilled or steamed vegetables or a piece of rye or wholemeal toast
Fish is delicious as well as quick and simple to cook, and provides your body with valuable nutrients. A poached fish fillet accompanied by a grilled tomato makes an excellent start to the day.

Uncooked breakfasts

Sugar-free cereal, such as flaked corn, with sunflower seeds
When you shop for a packaged cereal, check the ingredients label first to ensure that it does not contain any sugar. If you combine a serving of the cereal with some hazelnuts and sunflower seeds, topped with a tablespoon of live natural yoghurt and a teaspoon of sultanas, the cereal and sultanas will provide your complex carbohydrates and the nuts, seeds and yoghurt will supply your protein.

Nut and seed muesli
A simple recipe to mix up your own muesli (*see p.108*) should be one that includes whole grains, nuts and seeds to provide an ideal combination of the food groups.

BENEFICIAL NUTRIENTS

The best way to maximize your nutritional benefits is to eat as many unprocessed foods as possible. This is because the nutrient levels of, for example, whole grains remain intact as long as they have not been refined in any way. In contrast, the grains contained in processed cereals have been refined to such a degree that it's very possible the nutrient levels in these products are depleted.

So, when deciding what to eat for breakfast, remember that the fibre content and level of B vitamins in whole grains such as oats are potentially higher than those of processed cereals. In fact, oats contain most of the B vitamins, which have numerous functions in the body. These include being involved in the production of energy and in helping to maintain stable moods, which can, in turn, help to reduce your cravings for sugar and caffeine.

It may be worth making up a quantity of muesli in advance and storing it in a sealed plastic container ready for those mornings when you don't feel like doing anything more than pouring your breakfast into a bowl, adding some milk and eating it straight away.

Natural yoghurt with apple

For a tasty, quick breakfast, try mixing one chopped apple with two tablespoons of live natural yoghurt and sprinkling over a tablespoon each of flaked almonds and pumpkin or sesame seeds. The yoghurt, nuts and seeds provide the protein while the apple provides the complex carbohydrates and fibre. Turn to the recipe section for a similar recipe that includes fresh pear (*see p.107*).

Tofu smoothie

Try a smoothie for a change. Use a food processor to blend 50g (2oz) of soft tofu, one chopped apple and a tablespoon of either sunflower, pumpkin or sesame seeds with your preferred choice of full-fat milk – cows', goats', sheep's, rice or soya milk. Add a couple of drops of vanilla essence or a teaspoon of unsweetened cocoa powder if you like the taste, blend for a few seconds more and then drink the smoothie.

Try a **refreshing smoothie** made with **tofu, fruit and seeds** for a perfectly balanced breakfast

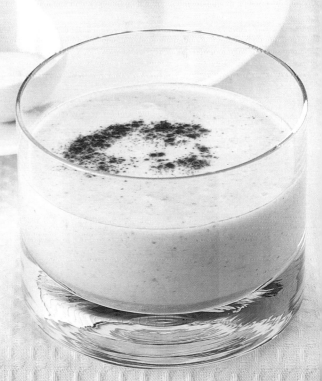

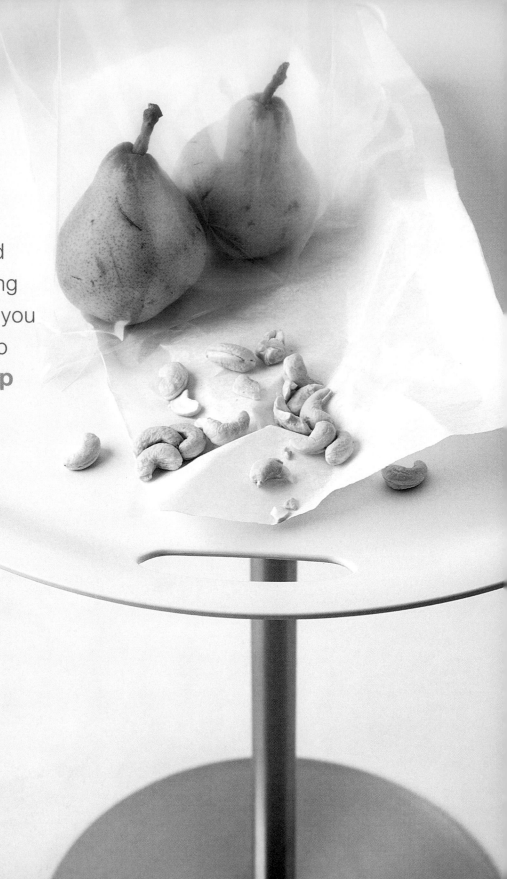

Ideally you need to **eat** something almost **before** you **feel hungry** so that you **fuel up** just before your **glucose** levels dip **too low**

Snacks

By the middle of the morning or afternoon, the energy created from your last protein-rich meal will have been used up by your body for various functions – anything from breathing and thinking to walking and exercising. At this point it's time to refuel again.

Assuming that you ate your breakfast at about 8am, you should eat a mid-morning snack between 10.30am and 11am. Likewise, if you ate lunch at 1pm, have a mid-afternoon snack at about 4pm. Ideally, you should eat something almost before you feel hungry so that you fuel up just before your glucose levels dip too low; don't wait until you feel ravenous.

Which snacks are best?

The snacks you choose needn't be a time-consuming culinary feast. For example, when I suggest eating some crudités and a dip, don't assume that you must cut the vegetables perfectly and arrange them artistically on a plate with the dip in the centre. You can just as easily stand in the kitchen, dip a carrot into an opened tub of dip and munch it. After all, it's the combination of the complex carbohydrate and protein that is important, not how it is presented. However you decide to eat your snack, do remember not to rush it and to chew each mouthful well.

If you go out to work, try to plan ahead by taking something simple with you in your bag, such as a tupperware box of chopped raw vegetables and a few cubes of hard cheese. You only need eat a few mouthfuls to make a satisfying snack.

Energy bars and drinks

Energy bars are not an ideal option. Many are sold as "healthy" but they are not as wholesome as they seem. Look at the labels of energy bars or drinks and you will see that they all contain sugar in varying amounts. Also check whether the protein content of an energy bar is anywhere near the correct Food Doctor ratio of around 40 per cent. Ideally, opt for the suggested snacks overleaf instead.

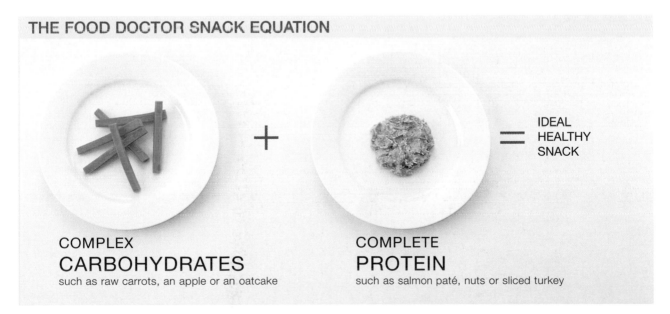

THE FOOD DOCTOR SNACK EQUATION

COMPLEX CARBOHYDRATES
such as raw carrots, an apple or an oatcake

\+

COMPLETE PROTEIN
such as salmon paté, nuts or sliced turkey

=

IDEAL HEALTHY SNACK

Snack suggestions

Snacking is an important element of the Plan for Life, and every mid-morning and mid-afternoon snack must include a combination of the right food groups (as the equation on the previous page shows). The timing of each snack is also significant, as are the amounts you eat.

If you take care not to leave too long a gap between your previous meal and your next snack, the chances are that you won't be tempted to overeat or make poor choices about what your snack should consist of.

Snacks should be easy and quick to prepare, although you may sometimes have to be a little creative with your ingredients. If you are out and about during the day, take a piece of fruit and a packet of mixed seeds or nuts in your bag – an apple and five nuts should make an ample snack. Even if you don't feel very adventurous about what to eat, make sure that your snack is healthy and simple to make, that it consists of the correct proportion of protein and complex carbohydrates and it is something that you enjoy eating.

TAKING SUPPLEMENTS

Although supplements can play a significant role in maintaining our health, I feel that many of us take too many of these products without knowing exactly what they do or how they interact. Since the Plan for Life is designed to enhance your digestion and improve the absorption of nutrients, I would prefer that your vitamins and minerals come directly from your food intake. There are one or two supplements that might make a small difference to your well-being, but most of your success will come from your dietary and lifestyle changes, not from a bottle of capsules. Rather than waste money on supplements that may not be necessary, make a one-off appointment with a nutritionist who will be able to tell you which supplements, if any, may suit your requirements.

Easy options

A piece of fruit with raw nuts

Choose an apple or a pear to eat with five or six Brazil nuts or almonds. Nuts make an excellent standby as you can buy them in small packets to keep at home or in your bag, briefcase or rucksack. It is important that you don't eat too many nuts – limit yourself to an average of five or six a day – and that you eat complex carbohydrates, such as a piece of fruit, at the same time. You may prefer to substitute nuts with a handful of mixed sesame, pumpkin and sunflower seeds. Soya nuts are now becoming widely available in shops and health-food stores, and, as they contain far less fat than other nuts, they make an excellent high-protein alternative. They may also be a good choice if you enjoy a little more variety.

Nut butter on two rice cakes, oatcakes, or a small piece of rye bread

Nut butters, such as peanut, cashew or almond butter, are another good standby, but ensure that the products you buy are free of sugar and that you don't eat too much at once. A thin scraping of your choice of nut butter on a rice cake, oatcake or piece of rye bread should suffice.

A tablespoon of dip with a few raw vegetables

Choose a dip such as guacamole, tzatziki, houmous or fish paste. If you would like to make your own houmous, see page 26 for a recipe. Chop up a couple of raw vegetables, such as a carrot, a stick of celery, some chicory, cucumber, a few broccoli florets or green beans, and use the pieces to scoop up the dip and eat it. If you go out to work, make things even easier for yourself by chopping up the vegetables at home first and storing the pieces in a sealed plastic bag. Keep the bag in a fridge at work if you can.

Guacamole on two oatcakes or rye crispbread

See page 134 for an easy recipe for homemade guacamole. If you add lemon juice to the ingredients when you make the dip, it will keep in the fridge for up to 24 hours.

Assemblies

Choose any **one** of the following complex carbohydrate bases:

**1 piece of rye toast or bread
2 oatcakes
2 rice cakes
2 corn cakes**

Top it with your choice of any **one** of the following protein sources:
Cheese – any type, although cottage cheese is the best choice. Avoid blue and aged cheeses.

Fish – a paté or spread made with any oily fish, such as mackerel, salmon, tuna or sardine.

Eggs – a chopped hard-boiled egg combined with finely chopped herbs such as parsley, dill or tarragon.

Chicken or turkey slices – use skinless poultry. If you buy pre-sliced products from the shops, ensure that they are sugar-free.

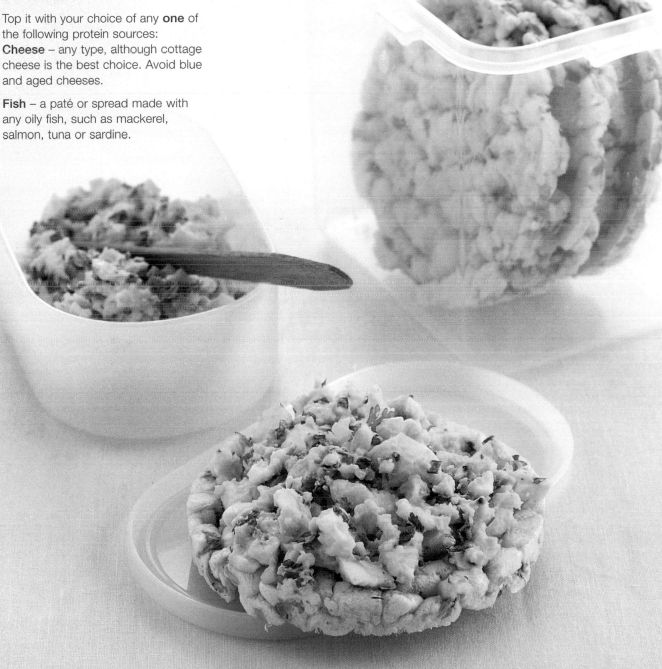

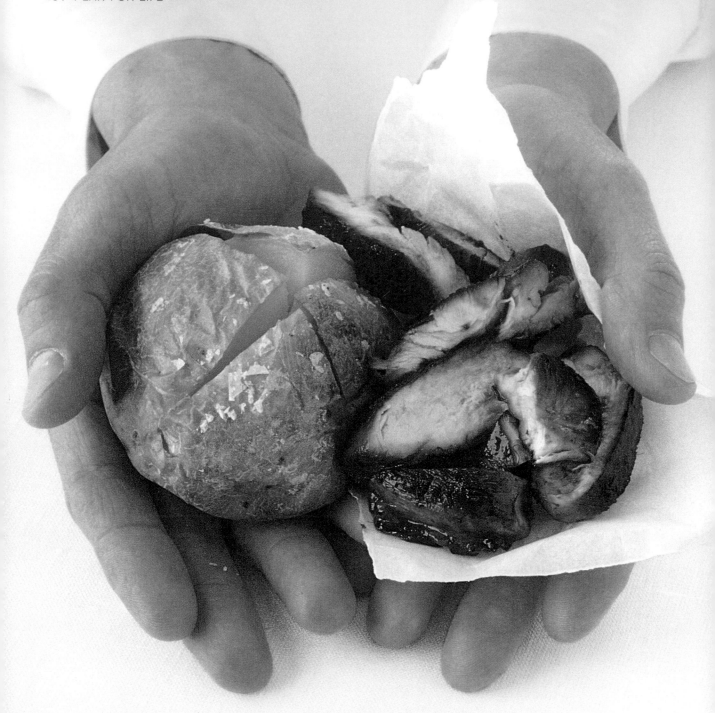

If you open your **hands** and **hold your palms** together, the **surface area** you see is the sort of **plate size** I have in mind

Lunch

When it comes to lunch, the most important thing to remember is that you should eat the right combination of complete protein, complex carbohydrates and fibre. The other rule to bear in mind is that you need to eat slightly larger quantities of food than you would at breakfast or dinner.

Your mid morning snack should have kept your glucose levels even until lunchtime, so at about 1pm it will be time to fuel up again. For this meal the quantities are slightly larger than those of breakfast or dinner, although it is important that you do not overeat.

How much do I eat?

If you hold out one hand and open it, the portion of protein you should eat is a little smaller than the size of your palm. Complex carbohydrates make up the remaining 60 per cent of the food on your plate. To gauge

how much food that should be, open out both hands and hold your palms together side by side – the surface area you see is the sort of plate size that I have in mind. As long as your food isn't piled too high, you should be eating more or less the right amount of food.

If you have the time and you enjoy cooking, then by all means make the effort to prepare your food; given that digestive enzymes respond to visual stimuli, this process can aid digestion. However, lunch doesn't have to be a beautifully prepared meal: you can easily cook a chicken

breast, or bring a cold, cooked piece of chicken in to work from home, and add a small jacket potato and vegetables or some brown rice salad. Not quite the visual feast you might hope for, but it can taste just as good and supply all the energy and nutrients you need through much of the afternoon.

If you usually buy sandwiches for your lunch, I suggest that you buy sandwiches for only two days of the week and prepare homemade lunches for the remaining days. Overleaf are some ideas for lunches to eat at home, at work and on the move.

THE FOOD DOCTOR LUNCH EQUATION

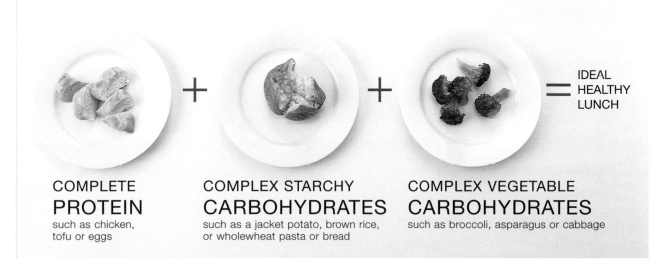

COMPLETE
PROTEIN
such as chicken,
tofu or eggs

COMPLEX STARCHY
CARBOHYDRATES
such as a jacket potato, brown rice,
or wholewheat pasta or bread

COMPLEX VEGETABLE
CARBOHYDRATES
such as broccoli, asparagus or cabbage

IDEAL
HEALTHY
LUNCH

Lunch suggestions

Lunch is often a potentially rushed and perhaps functional meal, especially if you are working or busy with your day. Yet however little time you have, it is vital that you put aside ten minutes or so to relax and eat your lunch calmly and slowly.

Taking just a short amount of time to eat your lunch properly and chew your food well will help to improve the process of digestion, thus allowing you to derive the maximum benefit from the good food you are eating. This process also helps you to reduce your stress levels in the middle of a busy day.

Away from home

For many people, lunch is the one meal of the day that is eaten away from home and if this is the case for you, it may help to organize in advance what you will eat so that your meals fit in with the Plan for Life programme. You might prefer to plan for the whole week, writing down a rough idea of what you intend to eat each lunchtime. Tie your lunch plan in with dishes that you will make for your evening meals so that you can cook extra quantities to take into work the following day. Here are some ideas to inspire you.

Meal options

Roast cod with pesto, steamed cauliflower and French beans
Lay the fish on a lightly oiled baking tray, spread a tablespoon of fresh pesto over the fish, season with freshly ground black pepper and roast in a medium-hot oven for ten minutes or so. See page 29 if you would like a recipe to make your own pesto.

Fresh soup with rye or soda bread
Make your own soup using lentils or beans and vegetables, or refer to the recipes on pages 23 and 123. Pea and ham or chicken and vegetable soup make a well-balanced protein and carbohydrate meal in a bowl.

One grilled turkey breast, tuna fillet or a hard-boiled egg
Serve with a salad that contains five different vegetables and salad leaves.

Chick-peas and sliced red pepper
Add pine nuts, a green salad and a salad dressing (see p.117).

Salade niçoise
Include your choice of tuna, black olives and green beans (see p.116).

Chicken Caesar salad
Mix pieces of cold, grilled chicken breast with a large green salad and a dressing (see p.117).

Goats' cheese salad
Add the cheese to a large mixed salad with a dressing (see p.117).

Smoked mackerel fillet
Serve cold with a large green salad and half a sliced avocado.

Mixed vegetable chowder
Using the recipe on page 124, substitute the fish and seafood with some diced fresh vegetables.

Mixed lettuce salad
Add sliced turkey, fresh asparagus and Feta cheese.

Poached or hard-boiled egg
Serve with a mixed bean and rice salad and sliced tomatoes.

Sardines, either fresh or tinned
Serve on rye toast with chopped dill.

One poached chicken breast
Serve with a mixed salad, roast vegetables or tabouleh (see p.113).

One small baked potato
Add a portion of tinned or fresh tuna fish, salmon, sardines, chicken or baked beans to provide the protein, and serve with a large mixed salad.

Sandwich selections

Choose **one** of the following breads:

Gluten-free
Wholemeal
Granary
Rye

Fill the sandwich with your choice of these proteins and some salad. Use minimal quantities of butter, mayonnaise and cream cheese:

Cheese – any type, although cottage cheese is the best choice. Avoid blue and aged cheeses.

Egg – use chopped fresh herbs as a flavouring instead of salt.

Chicken or turkey slices – use skinless poultry. If you buy pre-sliced products from the shops, ensure that they are sugar-free.

Smoked salmon – add a squeeze of fresh lemon juice for added taste.

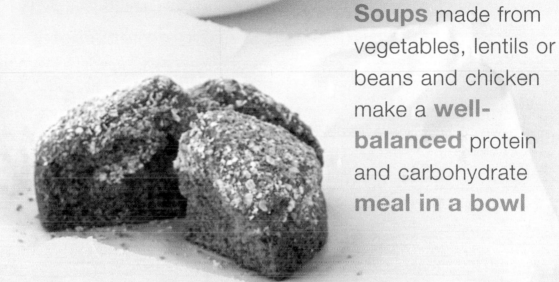

Soups made from vegetables, lentils or beans and chicken make a **well-balanced** protein and carbohydrate **meal in a bowl**

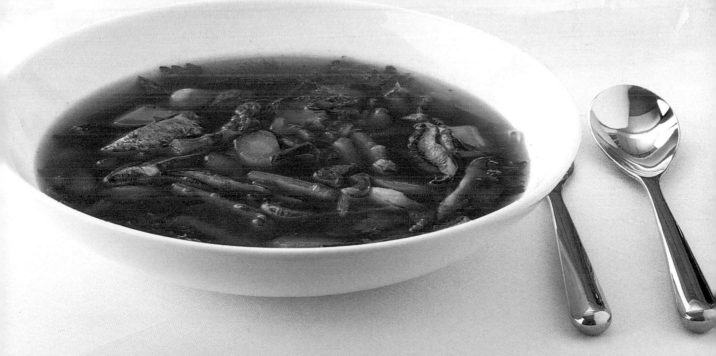

Choosing to **eat later** on in the evening, perhaps just a couple of hours before you go to bed, means that you should **omit starchy carbohydrates** and **increase** the complex carbohydrates from **vegetables** instead

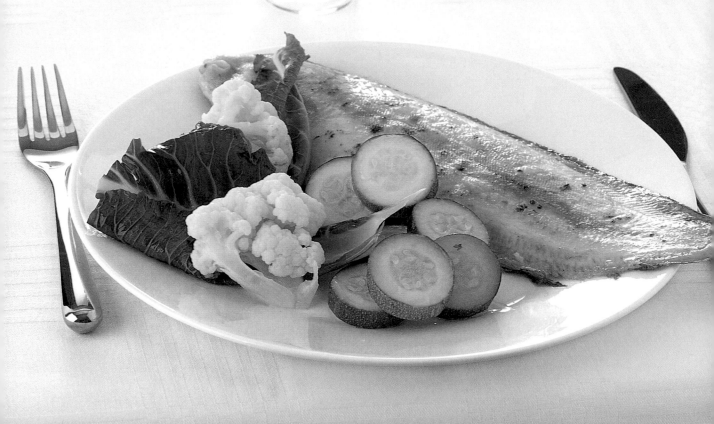

Dinner

In the modern world, dinner has become the main meal of the day. It's the one meal we don't have to rush and is usually eaten in the company of family or friends. This all means we have come to expect more from our evening meal than just eating to keep our energy levels even.

Breakfast and lunch are usually functional meals, but dinner is almost an event by comparison, especially if you eat together as a family or with friends. It is at this time that your good intentions to eat sensibly may falter or be forgotten entirely.

If your last snack was at 4pm, you should aim to eat dinner at 7–7.30pm. Try not to eat any later, but if you do then still eat a snack at this time – a few nuts and an apple or a raw carrot and houmous should be enough.

Many dieters will be familiar with the theory that carbohydrates, especially those containing grains,

should be limited in the evenings. It isn't necessary to avoid carbohydrates on The Food Doctor plan as long as you eat relatively early. However, if you choose to eat later on in the evening – perhaps just a couple of hours before you go to bed – omit the starchy complex carbohydrates and increase the amount of complex vegetable carbohydrates instead. This means that you include just protein and vegetables at dinner.

If you have an evening meal with family or friends and you can't adhere closely to The Food Doctor plan, go ahead and eat, but avoid

starchy carbohydrates containing saturated fats. For example, if your meal consists of steak, fries and salad, omit the fries and eat a large portion of salad and raw vegetables with your steak instead. This will make the meal healthier than it was, even though the steak contains saturated fat.

Plan ahead

Whatever you prepare, consider making a little extra for the next day. Cooking an extra chicken breast or another portion of fish at the same time will make your next meal or snack that much easier to prepare.

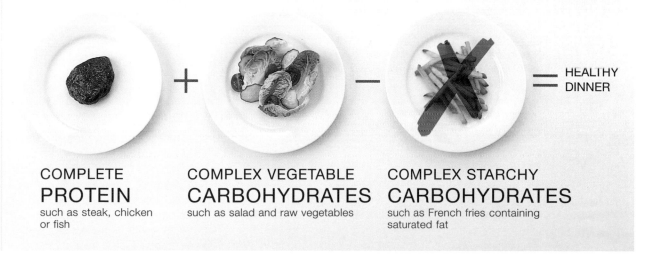

THE FOOD DOCTOR DINNER EQUATION

+   **−**   **= HEALTHY DINNER**

COMPLETE
PROTEIN
such as steak, chicken or fish

COMPLEX VEGETABLE
CARBOHYDRATES
such as salad and raw vegetables

COMPLEX STARCHY
CARBOHYDRATES
such as French fries containing saturated fat

Dinner suggestions

If you have time in the evenings and you enjoy preparing and cooking food, be as creative as you can with the meals that you eat. If time is short, however, or if your energy levels are low, then reach for store-cupboard ingredients or heat up some homemade soup from the freezer.

There are no prizes for guessing that, just like breakfast and lunch, dinner should combine protein and complex carbohydrates. If you eat your dinner later in the evening, remember to omit the starchy complex carbohydrates as you won't use the energy they provide.

First, select your protein. Choose from any one of the proteins listed on pages 50–51. These include cod, halibut, chicken, turkey or eggs.

Then choose your vegetables. It's all too easy to keep eating the same vegetables, so try to vary your selections (*see pages 52–53*).

Rather than flavour your food with salt, I suggest that you use herbs and spices to enhance the taste of your meal and make it more interesting (*see below*).

HERBS & SPICES

Food can taste very different depending on which flavourings you use. Try every herb you can, either fresh or dried, and select those you like best. Spices can also make a meal more interesting. Try not to overdo fermented sauces such as vinegar and soy sauce (which is also highly salted), and instead try a little teriyaki sauce.

Meal suggestions

Thai green chicken curry
Following the recipe on page 126, substitute the fish with one chicken breast and add some chopped fresh coriander leaves just before serving. Eat with lightly steamed vegetables.

Gingery roast vegetables
Select vegetables such as squash or pumpkin, Florence fennel, onions, tomatoes and courgettes, cut into chunky cubes and put in a shallow dish. Drizzle with olive oil and add a teaspoon of grated ginger. Roast in a medium-hot oven for 45 minutes and then serve with crumbled Feta cheese, goats' cheese or slices of mozzarella scattered over the top.

Mixed vegetable soup
Using the tomato and rosemary soup recipe on page 23 as a base, add pieces of raw chicken, fish, or a can

General – mint, marjoram, anise, cinnamon, caraway, rosemary, thyme, basil, sage, bay, nutmeg, sorrel, parsley.

Asian – lemon grass, chillies, coriander (seeds or leaves), garlic, lemon, pepper, ginger, sweet basil.

Indian – curry powder or paste, five-spice paste, garam masala, cumin seeds, cardamom pods, ginger, garlic.

of kidney beans or black-eyed beans when you pour in the stock. If you make fish or bean soup, prepare a larger batch and freeze extra portions.

Grilled Dover sole
Serve with green beans, steamed cauliflower and hollandaise sauce.

Whole roast trout
Place the cleaned fish in a shallow baking tray, season with freshly ground black pepper, add a knob of butter and scatter over flaked almonds. Cook in a medium-hot oven for 15 minutes or until the flesh is flaky. Serve with sautéed mushrooms and Florence fennel.

Spicy chicken
Mix a teaspoon each of ground coriander, cumin seeds, crushed garlic and water into a paste. Stuff the inside of a whole chicken with the spicy mixture. Drizzle over a little olive oil, season with freshly ground black pepper and roast the chicken in a medium-hot oven for one hour. Keep a portion of chicken aside for a cold meal the next day and serve the rest with grilled vegetables.

Mixed fish stew
See page 124 for a recipe. Serve with lightly steamed vegetables.

Baked mustard mackerel
Mix a tablespoon of sugar-free grain mustard with fresh lemon juice and spread it over the fish. Bake in a medium-hot oven for ten minutes or so. Serve with a green salad and fresh tomato relish (*see p.119*).

Quick options

Stir-fried tofu
Add freshly grated ginger, chillies and red and yellow peppers.

Stir-fried mixed vegetables with chicken or prawns
Stir-try the prawns or pieces of raw chicken first, then add chopped carrots, courgettes, asparagus, baby corn and herbs of your choice.

Roast asparagus
Place the asparagus in a baking dish, drizzle with olive oil and season with freshly ground black pepper. Cook for 10–15 minutes, then crumble Feta cheese over the top and serve.

Chick-pea and tomato stew
Use ingredients from your store cupboard for this recipe. Warm a can each of chick-peas and tomatoes in a medium-sized saucepan over a low heat and add chopped fresh or dried basil and parsley. Scatter pumpkin seeds over the top and serve with a selection of grilled vegetables.

Egg salad
Cut two hard-boiled eggs into quarters and serve with cherry tomatoes and a large green salad.

Greek salad
Combine fresh tomatoes, Feta cheese and black olives and serve with a large green salad.

Stir-fried squid
Prepare the squid according to the instructions on page 120. Stir-fry the chopped squid quickly in sunflower oil. Add chopped spring onions and pak choi and squeeze over fresh lemon juice just before serving.

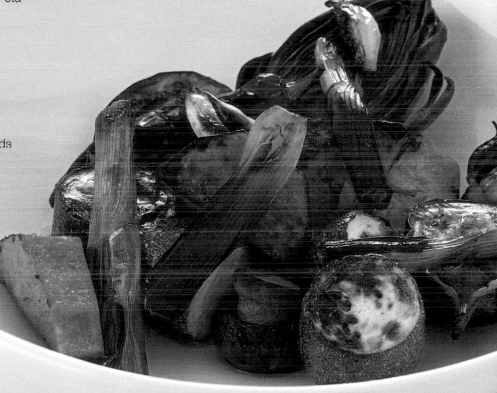

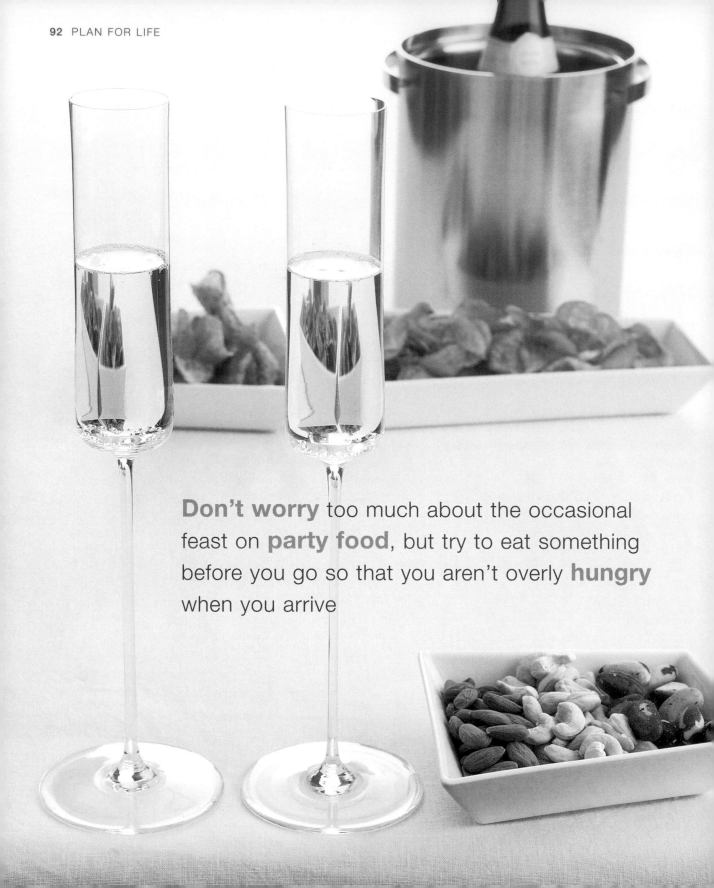

Don't worry too much about the occasional feast on **party food**, but try to eat something before you go so that you aren't overly **hungry** when you arrive

Special situations

Life isn't always predictable and, even when you know what your day is likely to hold, there will always be occasions when you will have to adapt The Food Doctor plan to work for you. Here are a few tips on how to cope with special situations and unexpected food choices.

Eating out

As long as you fully understand the principle of combining proteins with carbohydrates (see pp. 46–49), then eating out will be a lot easier than you may think.

The foods to avoid are those that are almost all pure carbohydrates, such as pizza, pasta, risotto, rice or noodles. For example, in a Chinese restaurant you could choose to order vegetables, fish and a little steamed rice rather than noodles and fried rice. This selection will help you to maintain a beneficial ratio of protein and complex carbohydrates.

Before you go out, it's a good idea to eat a small snack, even if it's just half a hard-boiled egg, to keep your glucose levels up so that when you come to order you aren't hungry enough to make poor food choices.

Finally, do be aware that restaurants use significantly more fat in dishes than you would use at home when making a similar dish.

Evening drinks

Going out for a drink straight after work can easily result in excessive alcohol intake, followed by a fatty, carbohydrate-loaded takeaway meal later in the evening. There is no reason why you shouldn't do this from time to time, but if it's become a regular occurrence then evenings such as these could be responsible for some of the increased weight that you want to lose.

The best way to minimize the damage is, as always, to eat a snack before you go out. Look at the suggested snacks on pages 82–83 for some ideas, but if you don't have time for a small snack then eat a few raw, unsalted nuts or olives with your drink and avoid all other bar snacks.

Parties

Party foods like savoury crackers and crisps are mostly simple carbohydrates, so they will soon leave you feeling hungry for more. But parties are to be enjoyed, so don't worry too much about the occasional party feast. Have a snack, such as a piece of rye bread with cheese, beforehand so that you aren't too hungry when you arrive. Eating this sort of snack also helps to reduce the rate at which your body absorbs alcohol – because once you have had too much to drink, who cares about losing weight?

On the move

If you are away from home all day and on the move, I suggest that you eat a substantial breakfast and have a packet of raw, unsalted nuts or seeds in your bag or briefcase to eat as your mid-morning snack. When it comes to lunch, have a sandwich by all means but buy one with added filling or discard half the bread to make one generously filled sandwich, so that the ratio of carbohydrates (in this case, bread) to protein (a filling such as meat or fish) is favourable.

Obviously it isn't always going to be easy, so the success of The Food Doctor plan depends on your ability to plan ahead a little. Make provisions for yourself so that you don't get caught in a situation where you have no choice but to eat the wrong foods. If this does happen – and of course it will sometimes – then just get back into line with the plan when you have your next meal.

Travelling

Whether you travel on a long aeroplane flight or take a short train ride, you may find it harder to eat food that fits easily into The Food Doctor plan. So, once again, try to plan ahead a little if you can.

If you are travelling by train, eat something before you leave the house. If the journey is a long one, you will probably need to take some food with you. A pot of houmous and some crudités in a sealed plastic container will make a convenient snack, while a wholemeal or rye bread sandwich generously filled with protein (such as tuna or egg) makes an easy meal.

A plane journey can prove more problematic. This may be one of those situations when you will have to accept that you just can't stick to your chosen food plan. If you are on a short flight, then you should be able to find something healthy to eat at the airport before you fly. If you are on a long flight, you may find that you are in luck and the main meal includes a lean protein. If not, don't worry about it, go ahead and eat what you are given and revert to the Plan for Life principles after you land. You can always take along a few apples and a packet of raw nuts such as cashews or almonds so that you can at least have a protein and carbohydrate snack as usual.

Holidays

Many people try to lose weight before they go on a beach holiday, only to put it all back on again while they are away. I am sure that most of us have heard people say to each other, "Go on, you're on holiday", and indulge in foods that won't do anyone any favours. Since The Food Doctor plan is a way of life, you shouldn't find yourself in this predicament. Many of my clients choose to follow the Seven-day Diet *(see pp.14–37)* before their holiday to ensure that they feel their best, and then eat sensibly while they are away.

If you are staying in a hotel that includes a continental breakfast as part of the room rate, you may have to invest in an extra breakfast dish to make sure you eat enough protein. Continental breakfasts consist purely of refined carbohydrates, and if you are intending to spend a lazy day on the beach you won't utilize the extra glucose generated by eating this kind of food. Instead, order eggs or cheese and a piece of bread or toast. This choice is far more likely to help you maintain your preferred weight during the holiday.

When it comes to lunchtime, limit your alcohol intake and ensure that you include some fish, meat or poultry in your meal. The same is true for dinner.

As it's likely that you will be eating your evening meals later than you would at home, it's a good idea to have some fruit – preferably hard fruits such as apples – available to keep you going. Keep a supply of raw, unsalted nuts too, but don't eat a whole packet at once.

You might also want to take some healthy snacks on long car journeys for yourself and any children travelling with you. A couple of plastic containers filled with a few slices of raw vegetables, grapes, cherry tomatoes and pieces of hard cheese should help them – and you – avoid the last-minute lure of fast food and all the unnecessary fats and sugars that these meals contain.

Eating with kids

Many clients tell me that they gain weight because they either pick at their children's food or eat with them at their favourite fast-food restaurants. It's all too easy to forget about fuelling up yourself while you worry about the kids and then suddenly feel hungry as they start to eat. As with all situations, it's best to plan ahead a little. If you pick the children up from school, eat a snack at home first, even if it's just a couple of mouthfuls or leftovers from your lunch. This will help you to resist the fatty, sugary foods that children seem to love. Alternatively, if you want to eat with the children, find something healthy that you can all eat: instead of burgers and fries, choose lean proteins, such as tuna or chicken, and some vegetables.

How do I cope with eating family meals?

If you have a family, think through your collective favourite foods, the sorts of dishes you make or buy that always go down well. Bearing in mind the principles of the Plan for Life, do such meals still fit in? Your family can continue to eat what they want, but you shouldn't forgo all of the foods that you have previously prepared to family acclaim.

Eating different meals to those of your family can sometimes create real problems, so the answer lies in which foods you leave out rather than what you replace them with. For example, if the family meal is pasta with a tomato sauce and vegetables, make sure that you have just a small spoonful of pasta and a much larger portion of vegetables. If you cook a roast chicken with all the trimmings, avoid the bread sauce and roast potatoes and enjoy the chicken and vegetables instead. You may have to make certain sacrifices, but your meals needn't be dull or unsatisfying.

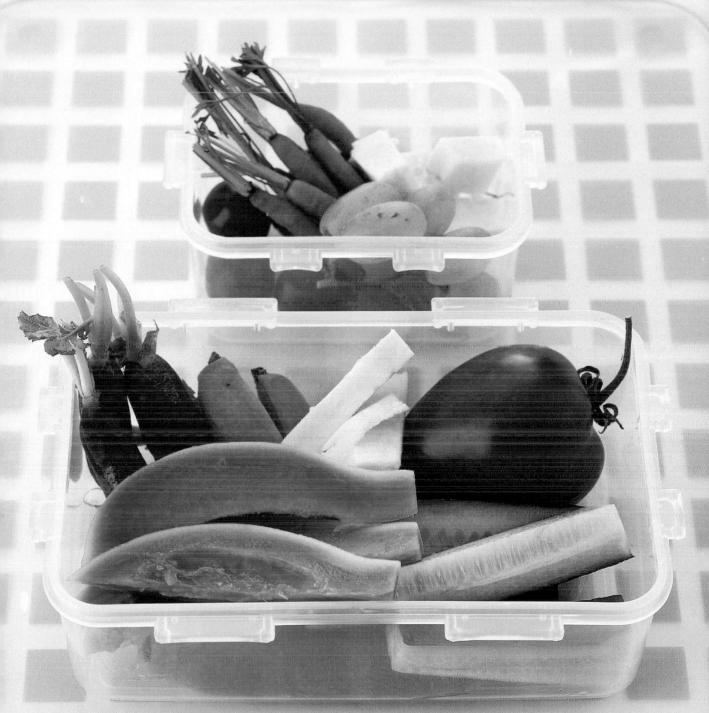

Take some healthy snacks in the car for yourself and your children when you travel to avoid the lure of fast food

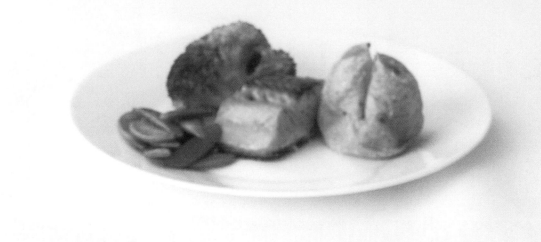

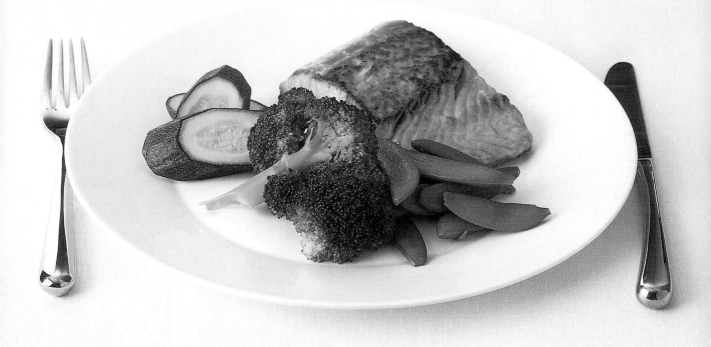

Nutrition quiz

Now that you have read through the Plan for Life, you have learnt about why I believe it is crucial to eat protein and complex carbohydrates in the right ratios. Hopefully, you now understand just what the implications are of combining the correct balance of foods for your health and well-being, and to aid weight loss. The challenge for you now is to put it all into practice.

Test your knowledge

It's now up to you to apply The Food Doctor plan to your own lifestyle. You will inevitably have to make quick decisions in everyday situations, so look back through the book again if you still feel unfamiliar with any of my principles. The Food Doctor plan is not complicated, but by understanding it correctly you will have a far higher rate of success. You can now try testing your knowledge of the ten principles by answering the simple questions in this interactive quiz.

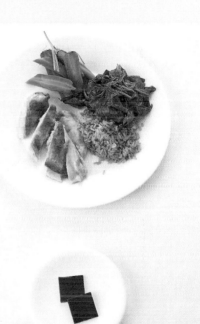

Do you remember the 80:20 rule *(see pp.68–69)*?

How knowledgeable are you?

Now that you have read the Plan for Life, put yourself in the following real-life situations to see if you know which are the best options to select.

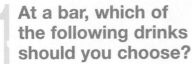

1 **At a bar, which of the following drinks should you choose?**

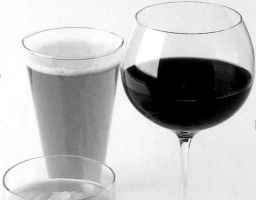

☐A glass of lager?

☐A glass of red wine?

☐A vodka and orange?

2 **Which is the best choice for a Food Doctor breakfast?**

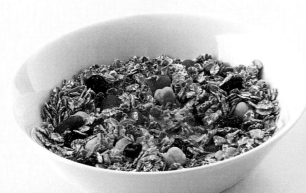

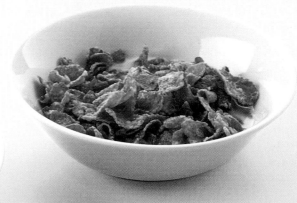

☐ Sugared cereal from a packet?

☐ Sugar-free muesli containing nuts and a small proportion of dried fruit?

3 **At a party, which of the following snacks should you choose?**

☐ Cocktail sausages?

☐ Crisps?

☐ Nuts?

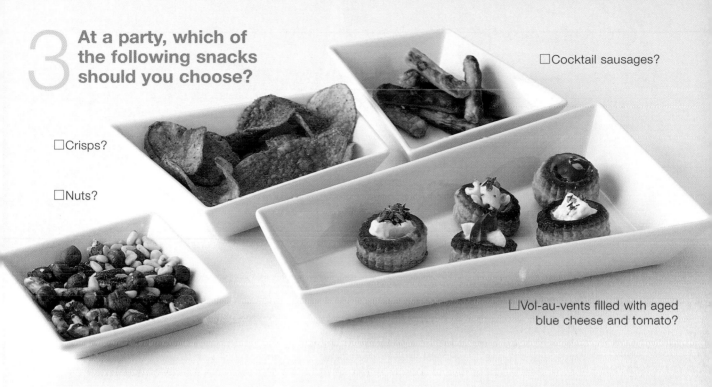

☐ Vol-au-vents filled with aged blue cheese and tomato?

4 **When in a restaurant, which of these meals would be best to choose from the menu?**

☐ Minestrone soup as a starter, mushroom risotto as a main course and passion fruit pavlova for dessert?

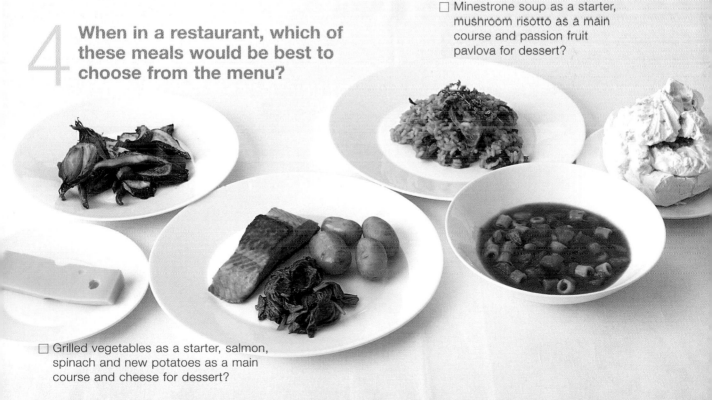

☐ Grilled vegetables as a starter, salmon, spinach and new potatoes as a main course and cheese for dessert?

5 **After exercising, which of these snacks should you choose?**

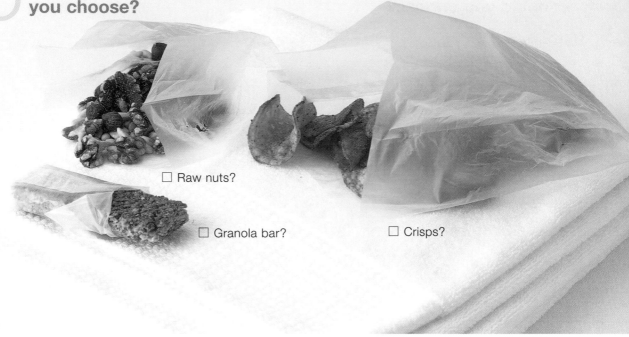

□ Raw nuts?

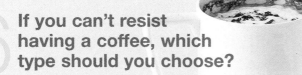

□ Granola bar?

□ Crisps?

6 **If you can't resist having a coffee, which type should you choose?**

□ Regular cappuccino?

□ Latte with skimmed milk?

□ Decaffeinated coffee with full-fat milk?

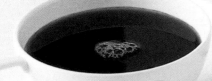

□ Black filter coffee?

7 **At a special occasion, which of these salad selections should you choose?**

☐ Pasta salad?

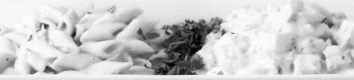

☐ Potato salad?

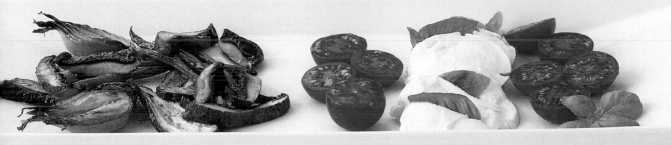

☐ Grilled vegetables?

☐ Mozzarella and tomato salad?

8 **At dinner, which of these meals should you choose?**

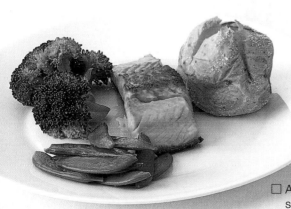

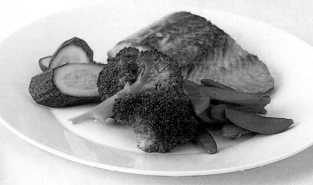

☐ A large portion of salmon and two large servings of vegetables?

☐ A portion of poached salmon, a small baked potato and a serving of vegetables?

How knowledgeable were you?

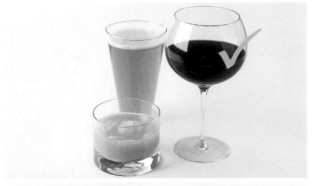

1 Red wine

While no alcoholic drink is ideal, red wine is the best choice as long as it is drunk with a meal or snack and not on its own. The vodka is mixed with orange juice – a simple carbohydrate – while the lager contains large quantities of yeast and sugars that encourage bloating.

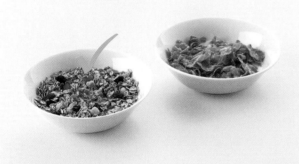

2 Muesli

The muesli is the best choice as it contains whole grains and nuts, both of which are converted from food to glucose fairly slowly.

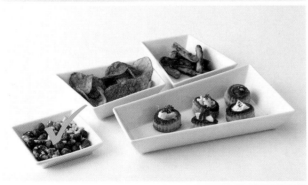

3 Raw mixed nuts

Although the nuts are rich in fat, they are the best choice because they contain no saturated fat. Had the vol-au-vents contained chicken instead of aged blue cheese and chopped tomato, they would have been the preferred choice.

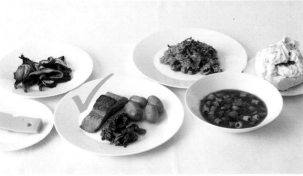

4 Grilled vegetables, salmon and cheese

The grilled vegetables provide some fibre, while the main course of salmon, potatoes and vegetables is almost an ideal meal: unlike the mushroom risotto, it supplies the right ratio of protein and complex carbohydrates. The cheese course should always include a small rather than large portion of cheese.

5 Granola bar

The granola bar will help to replenish the glucose that was spent while exercising. Such bars must contain some nuts, and as little sugar and honey as possible.

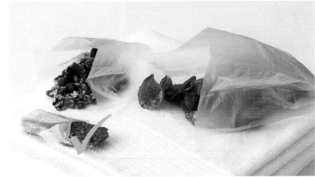

6 Decaffeinated coffee

While none of the options are ideal (you should not have more than 1–2 cups of coffee a day), the best choice is the decaffeinated coffee. Compared to the caffeinated versions, it is less likely to cause fluctuations in glucose levels, reducing the risk of food cravings.

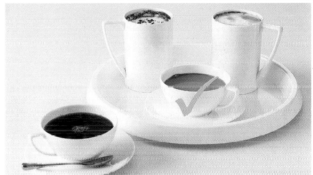

7 Mozzarella and tomato salad

Mozzarella cheese is a protein, while all the other salads contain only starchy carbohydrates. So the combination of cheese and tomato with a little olive oil provides a better ratio of protein to complex carbohydrates.

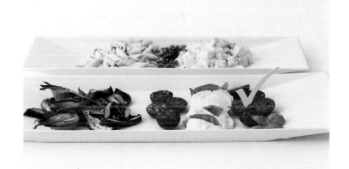

8 Both meals

These meals are both suitable choices as they contain the right ratios of food groups. However, the meal on the right would be most appropriate if you were to eat later on in the evening as it omits starchy complex carbohydrates in the form of the jacket potato.

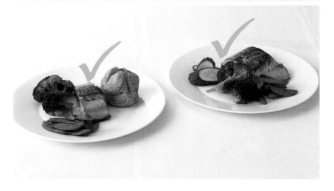

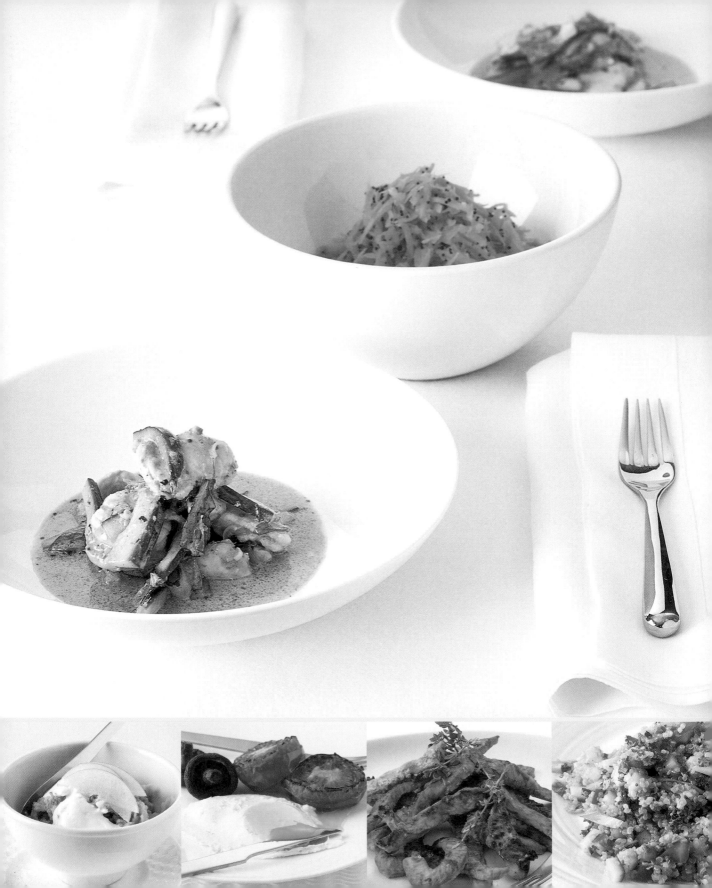

Recipes

Some of the recipes in this section are very basic and can be made in just a few minutes, while others need a little more preparation and cooking time. This will hopefully give you enough choice to suit your cooking skills and level of interest, and inspire you to try some new and original ideas. Remember that shopping for and cooking with the freshest, healthiest ingredients you can find are crucial to the success of The Food Doctor principles. For those of you who are still reluctant to cook for yourself, try the simplest of recipes to begin with. All recipes provide two servings.

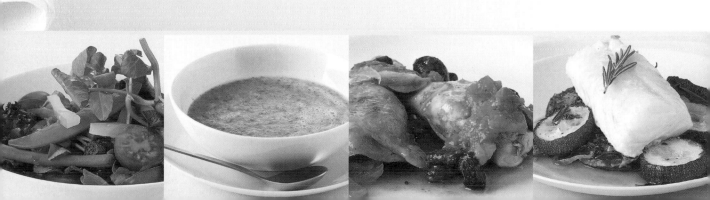

Hot apple oats

Oats are a good standby in your store cupboard, and they make a delicious, nutritious breakfast. Serves two.

4 tablespoons porridge oats
120ml (4½fl oz) water
1 apple
2 tablespoons live natural yoghurt

Place the oats in a small saucepan and pour the water on top. Leave the oats to soak while you grate the apple, reserving a few slices for a garnish at the end. Add the grated apple to the pan and cook the mixture over a low heat until simmering.

Let the oats cook for a couple of minutes more and then divide into two portions, each topped with a tablespoon of yoghurt and a few slices of apple.

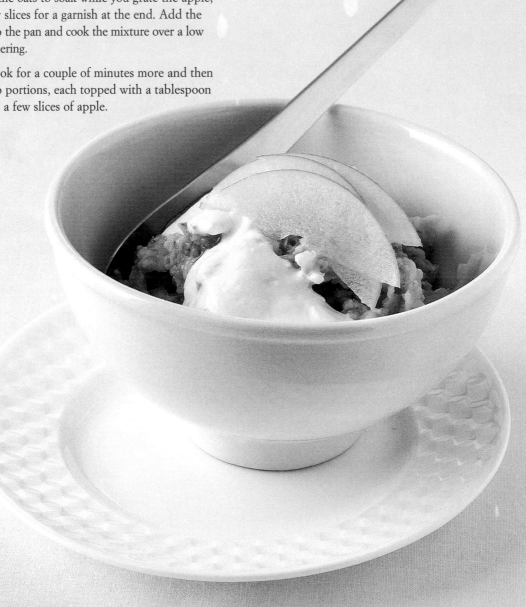

Yoghurt with fresh pear

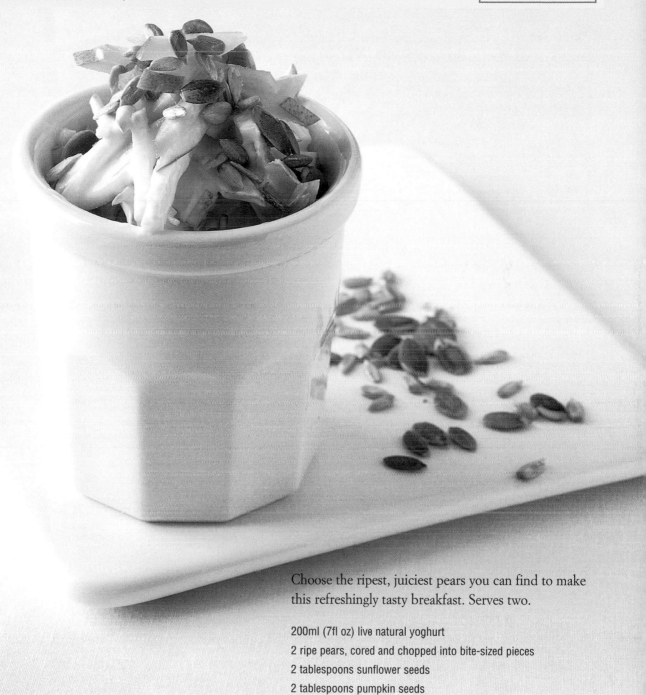

Choose the ripest, juiciest pears you can find to make this refreshingly tasty breakfast. Serves two.

200ml (7fl oz) live natural yoghurt

2 ripe pears, cored and chopped into bite-sized pieces

2 tablespoons sunflower seeds

2 tablespoons pumpkin seeds

Combine the yoghurt with the pear and divide into two portions. Sprinkle a tablespoon each of the seeds over the top of each portion and serve.

Nut-rich muesli

This muesli recipe has plenty of nuts for slow-release energy. To save time in the mornings, you can make a larger quantity and store it in an airtight container where it will keep for up to four weeks. Serves two.

1 flat tablespoon each of any **4** of the following:
barley flakes, rice flakes*, rye flakes, quinoa flakes*, oat flakes, buckwheat flakes*, millet flakes* (*gluten-free)

4 tablespoons mixed nuts, such as:
hazelnuts, cashew nuts, Brazil nuts, almonds, walnuts

6 teaspoons dried fruit, such as:
raisins, sultanas, dried apple rings (avoid very sweet dried fruit such as mango, papaya and pineapple)

2 heaped teaspoons mixed seeds, such as:
pumpkin seeds, linseeds, sesame seeds, sunflower seeds

2 tablespoons live natural yoghurt

120 ml (4½fl oz) milk (cows', goats' or sheeps' milk or an unsweetened dairy substitute such as rice or soya milk)

Mix all the ingredients together thoroughly and divide into two bowls. Serve each with a tablespoon of yoghurt and the milk of your choice.

Breakfast is the most **important** meal of the day as it boosts your energy to **optimum** levels

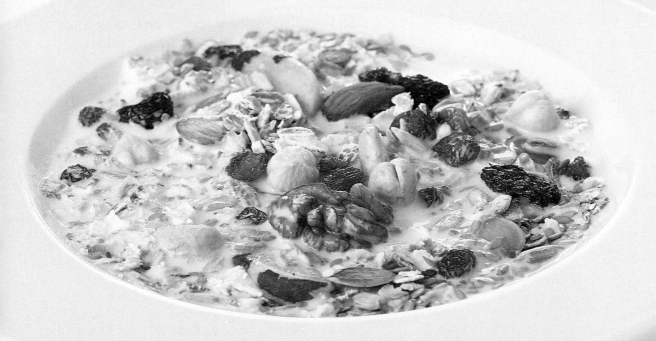

Breakfast berries

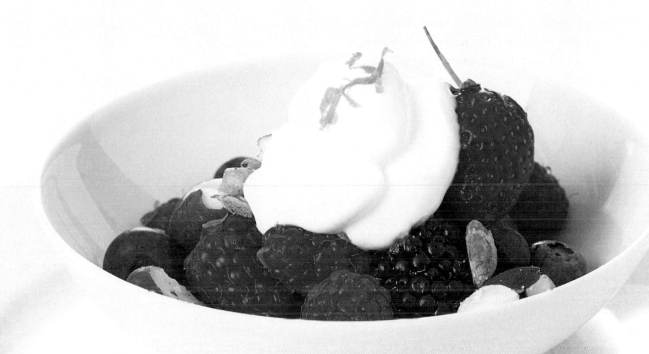

A **healthy** breakfast
will keep you **feeling**
satisfied for longer

Set yourself up for the day by relaxing for a moment with a bowl of juicy breakfast berries drizzled with fresh yoghurt. Serves two.

Juice and zest 1 orange

50g (2oz) each of any **4** of the following:
blackberries, blackcurrants, blueberries, grapes (halved and seeded), raspberries, strawberries

6 each of any **2** of the following:
almonds, Brazil nuts (chopped), hazelnuts, pistachios

2 tablespoons live natural yoghurt

Combine the juice and zest in a bowl, then add the fruit and nuts. Stir thoroughly and divide into two portions. Pour a tablespoon of yoghurt over each one and serve with a slice of wholemeal toast.

• For an exotic treat, substitute lime juice and zest mixed with a little fresh grated ginger for the orange, and tropical fruits such as papaya, pineapple and mango for the berries.

Baked salmon with fresh herbs

LUNCH OR DINNER

Cooking salmon in a parcel of kitchen foil helps to seal in the fresh flavours and keep the fish moist. If you only eat one portion of this dish, refrigerate the other serving and eat it cold the next day. Serves two.

200g (8oz) salmon fillets

Juice of ½ lemon

2 spring onions, finely sliced

2 tablespoons fresh dill, fennel and parsley, finely chopped

Preheat the oven to 180°C/350°F/Gas 4

Brush olive oil lightly over the centre of two large squares of kitchen foil. Place a salmon fillet in the middle of each piece of foil, skin side down, season with freshly ground black pepper, drizzle over the lemon juice and scatter the spring onions and herbs on top.

Seal the foil into a loose parcel by placing the ends together and folding them over several times, then transfer both packets onto a baking tray and bake for about 15 minutes.

When the fish is just cooked, but still pink inside, divide into two portions and serve.

SERVING IDEAS

For lunch Add a tablespoon of brown rice and a salad that includes a few diced, raw vegetables and your choice of dressing (see p.117).

For dinner Increase the salmon portions slightly and serve with large portions of vegetables. Omit the brown rice if you eat after 7pm.

Devilled turkey

This dish has a more intense flavour if you marinate the meat for up to two hours in the fridge first. The cooked meat will keep well for up to 24 hours in the fridge, but don't reheat it when you come to eat it for your next meal. Serves two.

200g (7oz) escalope or breast of turkey
1 tablespoon mustard
1 tablespoon Worcestershire sauce
A couple of drops Tabasco, more if you prefer a hotter dish

Cut the turkey into large strips. Combine the rest of the ingredients in a shallow dish. Add the turkey and let it marinate for at least 15 minutes, or preferably longer.

Remove the turkey from the marinade, cook it under a medium-hot grill for about 15 minutes, turning it occasionally, and then serve.

SERVING IDEAS

For lunch Eat hot or cold with half a small jacket potato, including the skin, and a mixed salad.

For dinner Increase the portion sizes slightly and serve with three different kinds of steamed vegetables. Omit the jacket potato if you eat later in the evening.

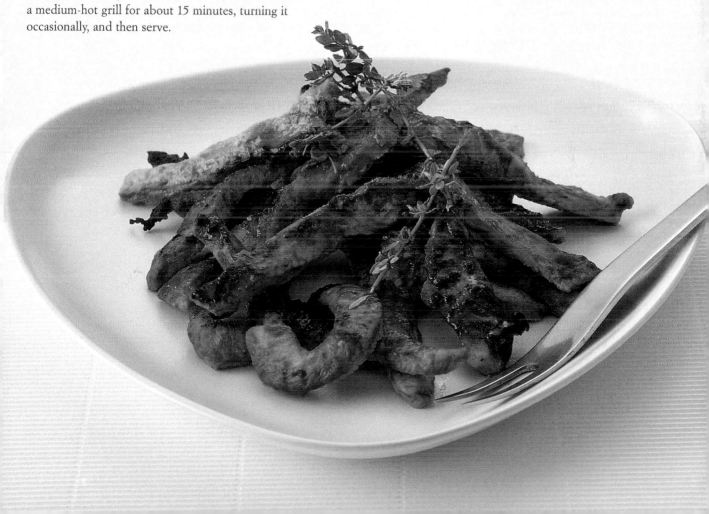

Oriental stir-fry

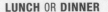

Stir-frying is a healthy option as you need only use a small amount of oil to cook your food. If you can't find these exotic ingredients easily, substitute them with other green vegetables and a larger quantity of brown mushrooms. Serves two.

SERVING IDEAS

For lunch Serve with a few rice noodles and some steamed bean-sprouts.

For dinner If you eat after 7pm, add more fibrous vegetables to the stir-fry and omit the rice noodles.

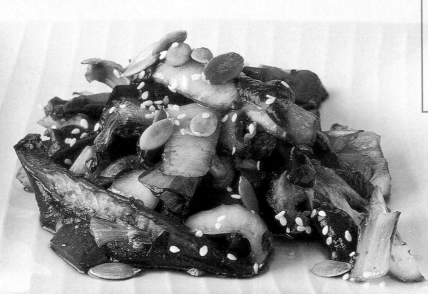

1 tablespoon soy sauce

1 teaspoon Thai fish sauce

1 teaspoon five-spice paste

1 teaspoon tomato purée

1 small clove garlic, crushed

250g (9oz) pak choi, stalks and leaves shredded

50g (2oz) large brown mushrooms, sliced

50g (2oz) mixed exotic mushrooms, left whole or sliced the same size as the brown mushrooms depending on the variety and size

1 tablespoon pumpkin seeds

1 teaspoon sesame seeds

Mix the soy sauce, fish sauce, five-spice paste and tomato purée together and leave to one aside.

Heat the wok gently, add a tablespoon of olive oil and soften the garlic. Turn up the heat and add the pak choi. Stir-fry for one minute until the leaves wilt.

Stir in the mushrooms until they are well coated with oil and beginning to soften. Add the sauce mixture, pumpkin and sesame seeds, stir well and serve immediately.

• To add the protein balance to this recipe, cut 100g (4oz) of either chicken, turkey or fish into strips and stir-fry for a couple of minutes before adding the pak choi.

• For a vegetarian alternative, cut 100g (4oz) of tofu into cubes and add that at the same time as the mushrooms.

Tabouleh

This recipe requires up to an hour of standing time, so prepare it well in advance of when you want to eat. It keeps for up to three days in the fridge. Serves two.

110g (4oz) couscous or bulgar wheat
600ml (1 pint) water
½ small cucumber, diced
2 medium tomatoes, diced and de-seeded
Juice of 1 lemon (about 3 tablespoons)
A small bunch each of fresh mint and parsley, finely chopped
1 tablespoon olive oil

Soak the couscous in the water for 30 minutes, then drain, squeezing out any excess moisture. Mix in the cucumber, tomatoes and lemon juice and season with black pepper.

Set aside for a further 30 minutes. Then add the herbs and olive oil, toss well and serve.

SERVING IDEAS
For lunch Add a tablespoon of tabouleh to your choice of protein and a mixed salad.
For dinner Have a small tablespoon as part of a main meal if you eat before 7pm. Omit this dish if you eat later in the evening.

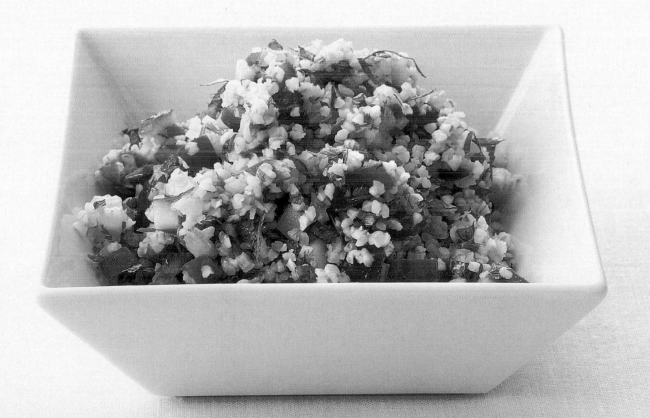

Tamarind chicken

Tamarind, the sticky pulp of the bean-like fruit from a tropical evergreen tree, has quite a sour taste, but with a hint of sweetness. Marinate the chicken for up to two hours before you cook it. Any leftovers can be stored in the fridge and eaten cold the next day. Serves two.

2 teaspoons tamarind paste

1 large clove garlic, crushed

1 teaspoon lemon juice

200g (7oz) chicken fillets

1 tablespoon fresh parsley, chopped

SERVING IDEAS

For lunch Eat hot or cold with a few new potatoes and steamed vegetables drizzled with a little walnut oil.

For dinner Increase the portion sizes slightly and serve with a salad or some vegetables. Omit the potatoes if you eat after 7pm.

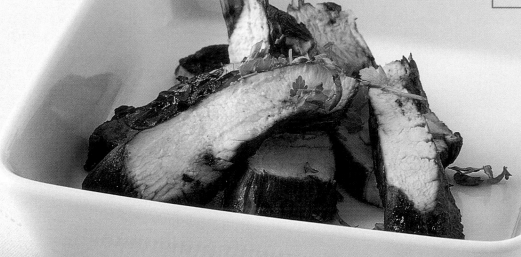

Combine the tamarind paste, garlic and lemon juice in a shallow bowl. Add the chicken and coat it in the mixture. Leave to marinate for at least 15 minutes, and ideally for an hour or two.

Remove the chicken from the marinade and place under a medium-hot grill for about 15 minutes, turning occasionally. Once cooked, slice into thin strips, scatter the parsley on top and serve hot or cold.

Fish fillet with lime

LUNCH OR DINNER

Choose the freshest fish you can find to give this dish the best flavour. Buy a small a packet of chick-pea flour and use it up quickly as it tends to lose its freshness after a short while. Serves two.

SERVING IDEAS

For lunch Serve with vegetables and a tablespoon of mashed potato.

For dinner If you eat later in the evening, omit the potato, increase the portion sizes slightly and serve with a variety of steamed vegetables.

200g (7oz) firm white fish fillets
Juice of ½ lime
1 large clove garlic, sliced
50g (2oz) chick-pea flour
1 tablespoon fresh parsley, chopped
½ lime, cut into wedges

Cut the fish into 2.5cm (1in) wide strips. Place them in a shallow dish, squeeze the lime juice over the top and season with freshly ground black pepper.

Heat three tablespoons of vegetable oil in a frying pan and warm over a gentle heat. Cook the clove of garlic for about five minutes, then discard.

In a separate shallow dish, sprinkle the flour in a thin layer, lift the fish from the juice, coat it in the flour and cook in the garlic-flavoured oil for one minute on each side until golden. Lift out the pieces with a slotted spoon, drain on kitchen paper for a few seconds and divide between two plates. Scatter with chopped parsley and lime wedges and serve.

Salade niçoise

LUNCH OR DINNER

This variation on a traditional salade niçoise, which also contains potatoes and anchovies, can be adapted to include your preferred choice of protein. Serves two.

SERVING IDEAS

For lunch Add a hard-boiled egg or a portion of tuna (fresh or canned) and a piece of rye toast to each serving.

For dinner Increase the portion sizes of tuna slightly, or divide three hard-boiled eggs between two servings, and omit the toast if you eat after 7pm.

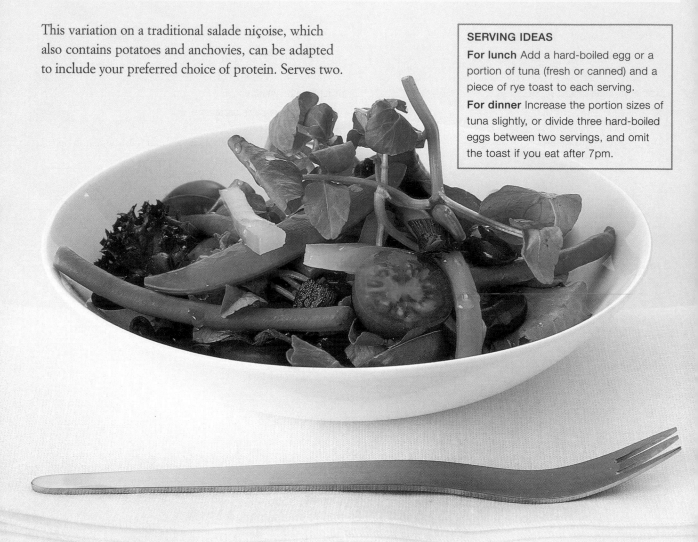

50g (2oz) green beans, cut into short lengths

50g (2oz) sugar snap peas or mangetout

A handful of frisee, oak leaf lettuce or curly lettuce leaves

6 cherry tomatoes, halved

½ yellow pepper, finely sliced

25g (1oz) brown mushrooms, sliced

6–8 pitted black olives

2 tablespoons cooked or canned red kidney beans

A few herbs such as basil, rocket or fresh fennel, chopped

Steam the beans and peas together for about 10 minutes until they are just cooked but still slightly crunchy.

Leave the vegetables to cool while you tear the lettuce leaves and arrange them in a salad bowl. Layer the salad with the remaining ingredients, scattering the fresh herbs over the top.

Pour over a simple French dressing *(see opposite page)* and toss the ingredients well just before serving with your choice of protein.

Salad dressings

Simple French dressing

2 tablespoons olive oil

1 teaspoon cider vinegar

½ teaspoon Dijon mustard

Combine the ingredients well using a small hand whisk and season with freshly ground black pepper. Keep the dressing in the fridge for a maximum of one week.

Oriental dressing

3 tablespoons olive oil

1 tablespoon soy sauce

1 tablespoon lime juice

½ teaspoon five-spice paste

Mix the ingredients well using a small hand whisk. This dressing can be kept in the freezer for up to one month.

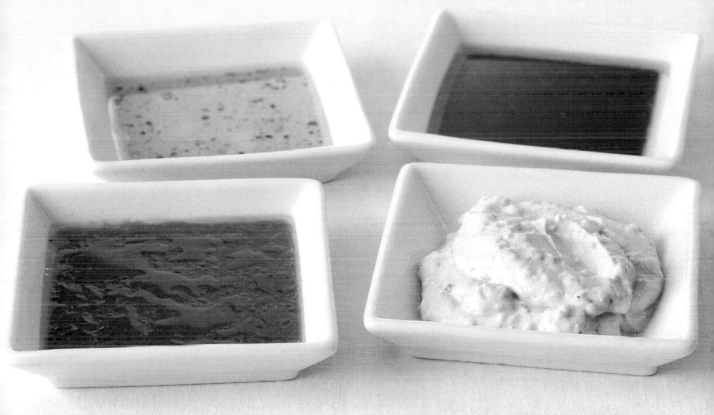

Vegetable juice dressing

100ml (4oz) organic vegetable juice

50ml (2fl oz) lemon juice

50ml (2fl oz) olive oil

Blend the ingredients well using a small hand whisk and season with freshly ground black pepper. If you want more punch to this dressing, add one crushed clove of garlic. This dressing freezes well for up to one month.

Avocado dressing

1 ripe avocado

220g (8oz) live natural yoghurt

Stone and peel the avocado. To retain some texture in the dressing, use a fork to roughly mash the avocado with the yoghurt. Season with freshly ground black pepper and keep the dressing in the fridge for up to 24 hours.

Simple chick-pea purée

With its creamy taste and nutty aroma, this chick-pea purée forms a nutritious and versatile protein choice. It keeps well in the fridge for up to three days. Serves two.

400g (14oz) can chick-peas, drained and well-rinsed

2 sprigs fresh thyme or ½ teaspoon dried thyme

1 large clove garlic

3 generous tablespoons live natural yoghurt

Put the chick-peas, thyme and garlic into a small pan and cover with water. Bring to the boil and simmer gently for 15 minutes.

Drain the chick-peas, tip them into a bowl and lift out the fresh thyme. Add the yoghurt and mash by hand for a coarse purée, or mix in a blender for a smoother texture.

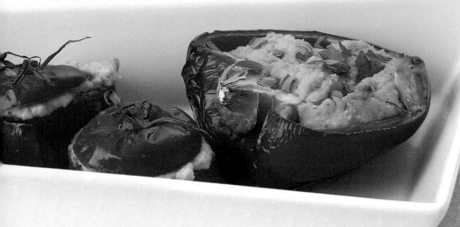
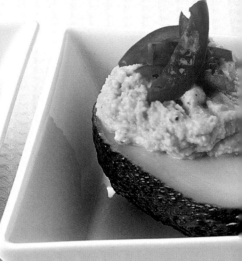

Vegetables stuffed with chick-pea purée

4 tablespoons chick-pea purée

2 tablespoon fresh parsley, chopped

A squeeze of lemon juice and a little lemon zest for added taste

2 large red or yellow peppers, halved and de-seeded, or 4 medium tomatoes with the tops cut off and pulp removed

Preheat the oven to 180°C/350°F/Gas 4.

Mix the purée, parsley, lemon juice and zest. Fill the pepper or tomatoes with purée, place on a baking dish, season with black pepper and drizzle with olive oil. Cover in foil and bake for 30 minutes. Serve with a dressed mixed leaf salad.

Avocado stuffed with chick-pea purée

2 tablespoons chick-pea purée

A squeeze of lemon juice and a little lemon zest for added taste

1 ripe avocado

1 tomato, chopped

Mix the chick-pea purée with the lemon juice and zest and season with freshly ground black pepper to taste.

Cut the avocado in half, lift out the stone and fill the centres with the purée. Serve each half on a plate with the chopped tomato scattered across the top.

Falafel

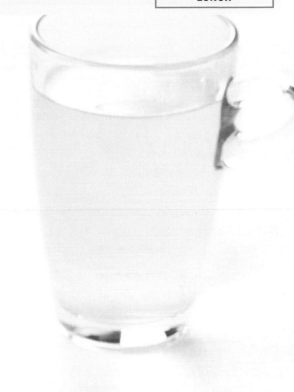

These spicy Moroccan chick-pea burgers can be eaten hot or cold, and will keep in the freezer for up to one month. Serves two.

400g (14oz) can chick-peas, drained and well-rinsed

1 large clove garlic

1 small onion, chopped

1 teaspoon ground coriander

1 teaspoon ground cumin

1 heaped tablespoon buckwheat flour

2 medium tomatoes, roughly chopped and mixed with the juice of 1 lemon and a drizzle of olive oil

200g (7oz) live natural yoghurt mixed with ½ teaspoon each of cayenne pepper and turmeric powder

Blend the chick-peas, garlic, onion and spices in a food processor until almost smooth. Scrape the paste into a bowl and mix in the flour. Divide into eight balls, each about the size of a golf ball. Flatten into patties (or baby-burgers).

Heat a tablespoon of olive oil in a frying pan and gently brown the falafels on each side – they should all fit in at once. Add a little more oil, if needed, when you turn them.

Serve the falafel with the tomato relish and yoghurt mix.

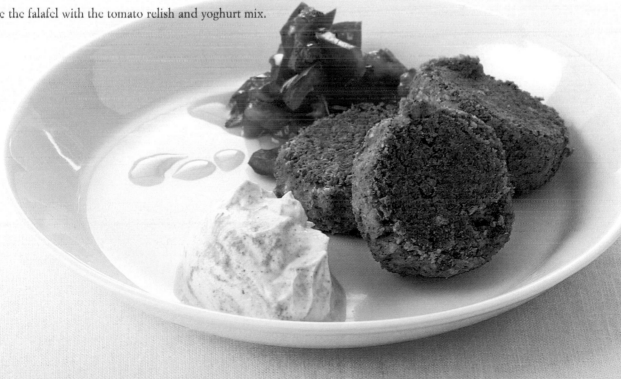

Squid in a fresh tomato sauce

Squid is easy to prepare, but you can ask a fishmonger to cut and clean it for you, or buy it pre-cleaned. If you want to make extra portions, this dish can be frozen for up to one month and then reheated gently. Serves two.

500g (16oz) squid
1 medium onion, chopped
1 large clove garlic, crushed
250g (9oz) tomatoes, peeled and diced
1 tablespoon lemon juice, and a little lemon zest for added taste
¼ teaspoon saffron threads, crushed in a spoon with a little water
A generous handful of fresh parsley and coriander, chopped

To prepare the squid, pull the head from the sac to draw out the innards and spine. Scrape off the pinkish outside membrane from the sac, rinse the sac and cut into rings. Sever the tentacles from the head, cut into pieces and rinse.

Soften the onion in a little olive oil in a small pan, then add the garlic and stir for two minutes. Add the tomatoes, lemon juice, zest and saffron. Stir in the squid and pour in just enough water to cover it. Simmer for five minutes until the squid is opaque but not rubbery.

Stir in the herbs and serve with a spoonful of brown rice and a green salad with an olive oil and lemon dressing.

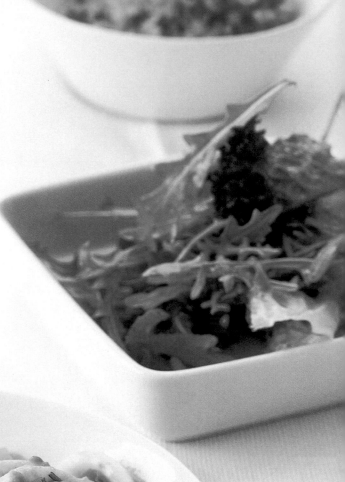

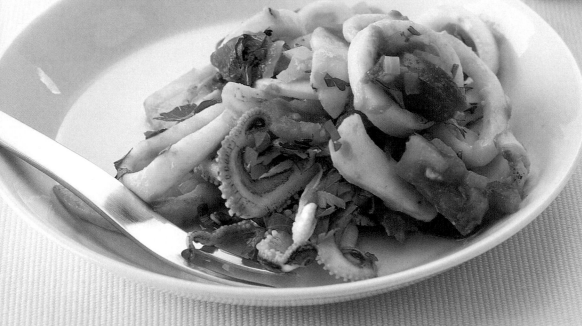

Tabouleh South American style

Keep this salad in an airtight container in the fridge for up to three days and serve a spoonful of it with a portion of chicken or fish. Serves two.

120g (4oz) quinoa

250ml (8fl oz) water, with a pinch of bouillon powder added

½ cucumber, diced

2 medium tomatoes, diced

2 spring onions, finely sliced

Juice of ½ lemon

A small bunch each of fresh mint and parsley, finely chopped

1 tablespoon olive oil

Gently simmer the quinoa and water in a small pan for 15 minutes or so until all the water is absorbed.

Meanwhile, chop the remaining ingredients. Once the quinoa has cooled, stir in the vegetables. Transfer to a bowl and allow to stand in the fridge for 10–15 minutes to let the flavours develop. Drizzle over the olive oil, season with freshly ground black pepper and serve.

Always serve a **small portion** of starchy carbohydrates with protein and vegetables at lunchtime

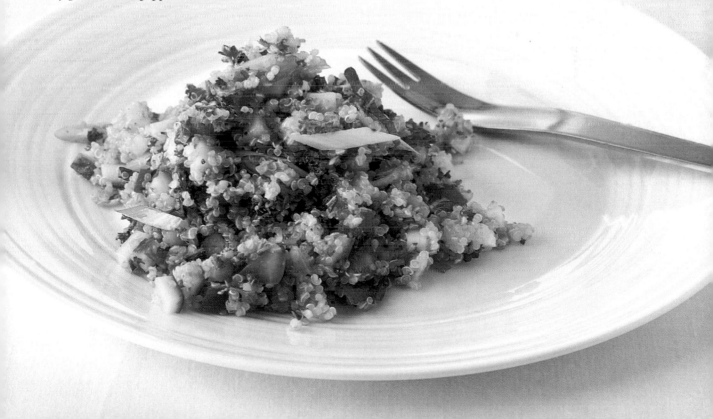

Pipérade

A wonderfully simple dish to prepare and cook, pipérade should be eaten immediately while it is still piping hot. Serves two.

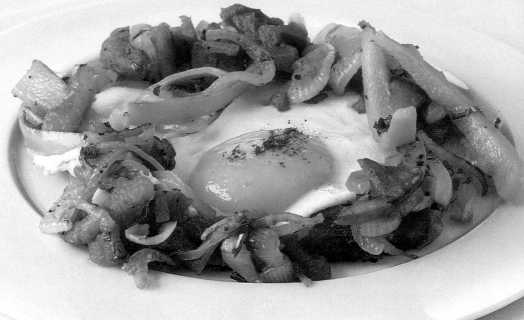

1 small onion, sliced

1 yellow pepper, de-seeded and cut into strips

2 medium tomatoes, peeled and sliced

A pinch cayenne pepper

1 tablespoon fresh mint, chopped

2 large eggs

Soften the onion and pepper in two tablespoons of olive oil in a frying pan over a low heat until the onion slices are golden. Add the tomatoes, cayenne pepper and mint and stir for a minute or two.

Either break the eggs on top of the vegetables or beat them first and add them to the pan so they cook like scrambled eggs. Cook gently until the eggs are set and then serve.

Watercress and carrot soup

This recipe is worth freezing if you want to save your second serving or make up a larger batch of individual portions to defrost another time. Serves two.

1 small onion, chopped

250g (9oz) carrots, chopped

1 bunch fresh watercress

1 small can chick-peas or ½ large can chick-peas

750ml (1pint) fresh vegetable stock; or add 1 tablespoon yeast-free bouillon powder to 750ml (1pint) water

1 teaspoon ground cumin

Gently heat a tablespoon of olive oil in a medium-sized saucepan and soften the onion. Add the chopped carrots and soften for five minutes.

Chop the watercress straight into the pan, stalks and all – this is easily done using a pair of scissors. Stir well until the watercress is mixed in and beginning to wilt. Add the chick-peas, stock and cumin and simmer gently for 20 minutes or so until the carrots are just cooked.

Blend the soup in a processor until smooth, season with freshly ground black pepper to taste and serve.

The Food Doctor soups are full of **nutrients** and can easily be augmented with extra protein for a **delicious** meal

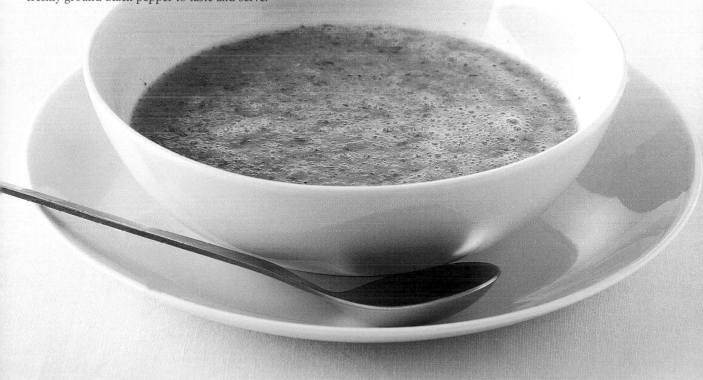

Easy fish chowder

This soup is more like a stew and is full of nutrients. Buy ready-made fresh stock from a good supermarket for this recipe as dried fish cubes are too salty. Freeze any extra portions, then defrost and gently reheat them as required. Serves two.

100g (4oz) white fish fillet, cut into bite-sized chunks

Juice of ½ lemon

100g (4oz) onion, chopped

2 large cloves garlic, crushed

500ml (1 pint) fresh fish stock

3 medium tomatoes, skinned and chopped

1 bay leaf

100g (4oz) cooked mixed seafood

75g (3oz) canned flageolet beans, drained

1 tablespoon each fresh coriander, parsley and dill, chopped

Marinate the fish in the lemon juice while you prepare the rest of the ingredients.

Soften the onion and garlic in a tablespoon of olive oil over a low heat in a medium-sized saucepan. Add the stock, tomatoes, bay leaf and white fish. Simmer very gently for about five minutes.

Add the seafood and flageolet beans and simmer for two minutes more until the seafood has heated through thoroughly. Season with freshly ground black pepper, stir in the herbs and serve.

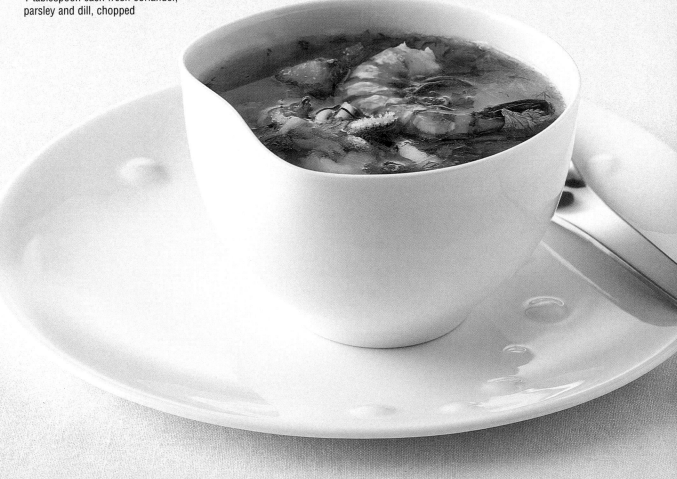

Garlic broccoli with Feta cheese

If you tend to find Feta cheese very salty, rinse the block of cheese under cold running water first before you cube it. Serves two.

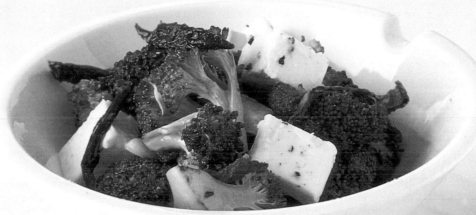

100g (4oz) Feta cheese, cut into small cubes

2 teaspoons lemon juice

2 teaspoons olive oil

Several sprigs fresh parsley, chopped

1 clove garlic, crushed or finely chopped

250g (9oz) broccoli, cut into small florets

50g (2oz) sun-dried tomatoes, cut into thin strips

Marinate the Feta cheese in the lemon juice, olive oil, chopped parsley and a seasoning of freshly ground black pepper while you cook the broccoli.

Gently heat a tablespoon of olive oil in a frying pan, add the garlic and cook for one minute. Then add the broccoli and sun-dried tomatoes and stir occasionally until the broccoli is tender but with a little bite left in it.

Lift the Feta cheese out of the marinade with a slotted spoon and add to the frying pan. Gently stir the ingredients and serve with the remains of the marinade poured on top.

Monkfish curry with carrot salad

DINNER

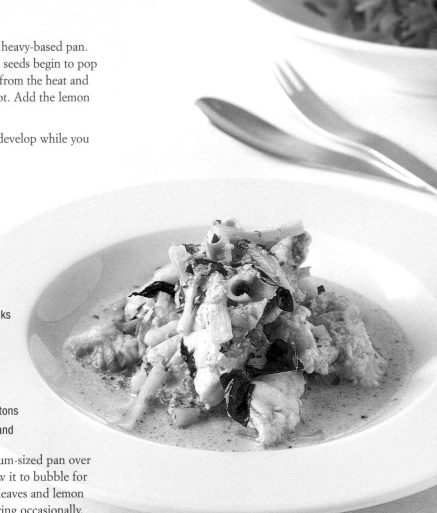

The monkfish in this recipe can be substituted with another firm, white fish such as cod or haddock, or even strips of chicken breast if you prefer. Serves two.

Salad

1 heaped teaspoon black mustard seeds

120g (4oz) carrots, grated

1 teaspoon lemon juice

Heat a tablespoon of olive oil in a small, heavy-based pan. Once hot, add the mustard seeds. As the seeds begin to pop (it only takes a few seconds), lift the pan from the heat and pour the oil and seeds over the raw carrot. Add the lemon juice and toss.

Leave to cool and allow the flavours to develop while you cook the monkfish.

Curry

1 tablespoon green curry paste

250g (9oz) monkfish, cut into bite-sized chunks

2 or 3 kaffir lime leaves, torn

1 stalk lemon grass, bruised and chopped

120ml (4½fl oz) canned coconut milk

1 tablespoon Thai fish sauce

½ small cucumber, de-seeded and cut into batons

A dozen or so basil leaves, torn roughly by hand

Heat a tablespoon of olive oil in a medium-sized pan over a low heat, add the curry paste and allow it to bubble for a minute or so. Add the monkfish, lime leaves and lemon grass. Cook gently for two minutes, stirring occasionally.

Stir in the coconut milk and simmer for five minutes or so until the fish is tender. Stir in the fish sauce, cucumber and the basil leaves and serve with the carrot salad.

Hot and sour chicken salad

You need to think a couple of hours ahead with this recipe to allow enough time to let the chicken marinate and the flavours develop properly. Serves two.

1 large chicken breast fillet, skinned and sliced thinly

For the marinade:
1cm (½in) fresh ginger root, peeled and grated

1 small clove garlic, chopped

2 teaspoons crunchy peanut butter

1 tablespoon fresh coriander, chopped, plus extra to garnish

1 tablespoon cider vinegar

1 teaspoon Thai fish sauce

1 tablespoon olive oil

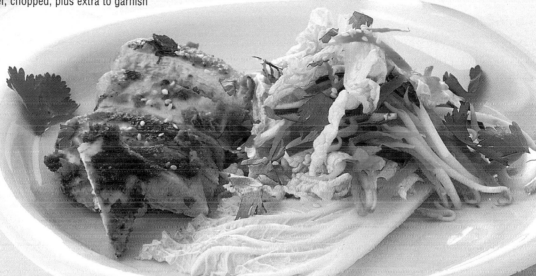

Salad

100g (4oz) bean-sprouts

50g (2oz) Chinese leaves, shredded

1 medium carrot, cut into sticks

1 small red onion, finely sliced into rings

1 teaspoon sesame seeds

Combine the marinade ingredients in a small bowl, add the chicken pieces and leave them to marinate for a couple of hours in the fridge.

Heat a tablespoon of olive oil in a wok over a high heat, remove the chicken from the marinade and stir-fry it for five minutes or so.

Mix together the salad ingredients and arrange on two plates. Transfer the chicken to the plates, scatter with sesame seeds and chopped coriander and serve immediately.

Leek and quinoa risotto

DINNER

Serve this dish with a crisp green salad, tossed in your choice of dressing *(see p.117)*, to offset the soft texture of the leeks and quinoa. Extra portions can be frozen for up to one month, then reheated. Serves two.

2 small leeks, about 200g (7oz)

250ml (8fl oz) water, with a good pinch of bouillon powder added

50ml (2fl oz) olive oil

1 tablespoon tomato purée

100g (4oz) quinoa

100g (4oz) portabello mushrooms, thickly sliced

2 teaspoons ground coriander

1 tablespoon fresh parsley, chopped

Juice of ½ lemon

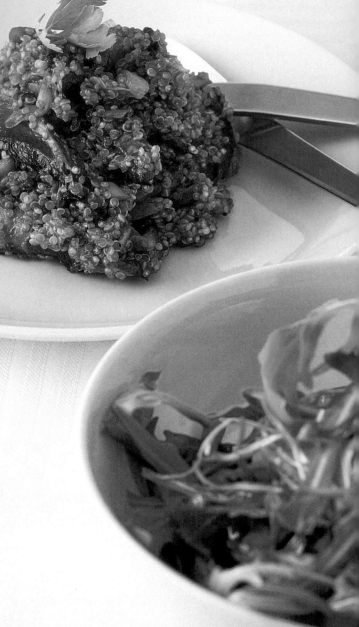

Slice the white parts of the leeks only into 1cm (½in) rings and rinse well. Pour the water and oil into a medium-sized saucepan, add the leeks and tomato purée and bring to the boil. Simmer for five minutes, then add the quinoa, mushrooms and coriander.

Simmer for a further 15 minutes or so until the water is absorbed. Stir in the parsley and lemon juice, season with freshly ground black pepper and serve with a green salad.

Lentils with fresh ginger

To make cardamom seeds into a powder, simply split several cardamom pods with a small, sharp knife, tip the seeds into a pestle and mortar and grind them up.

150g (5oz) dried lentils

250ml (8fl oz) vegetable stock

1 small onion, chopped

1 clove garlic, crushed

2cm (¾in) fresh ginger root, grated

1 teaspoon cardamom seeds, ground to a powder

3 large ripe tomatoes, skinned and chopped

2 tablespoons fresh coriander leaves, chopped

1 tablespoon sunflower seeds

Bring the lentils and stock to the boil in a medium-sized pan and simmer over a low heat for 30 minutes until the lentils are soft. Drain the lentils and leave to one side.

In the same pan, soften the onion and garlic in a tablespoon of olive oil over a low heat. Stir in the ginger, cardamom and almost all the tomatoes, keeping some back for a garnish. Cook for a few minutes.

Return the lentils to the pan and season with freshly ground black pepper. Heat thoroughly, turn out onto two plates, top with sunflower seeds and chopped coriander and serve with a mixed leaf salad.

Freeze dishes such as this to **build up** a stock of nutritious, instant **meals**

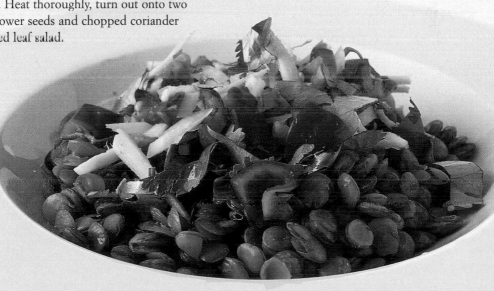

Fish with roasted vegetables

Any firm, white fish steak or fillet is suitable for this recipe. Ensure that you don't over-cook the fish as the flavour will be impaired. Serves two.

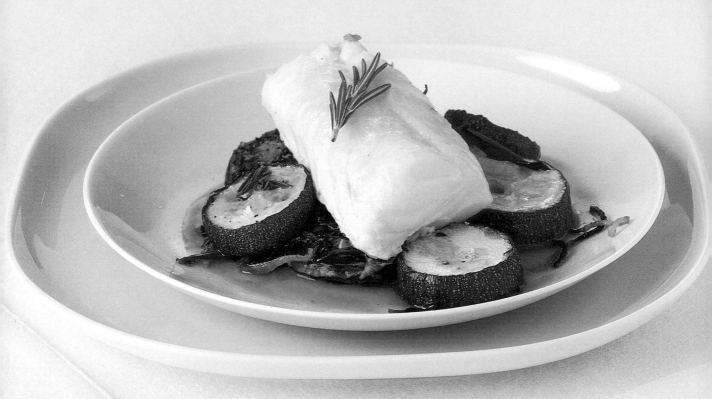

400g (15oz) white fish steak or fillet, such as haddock or cod, skinned

A squeeze of lemon juice

200g (7oz) courgettes, cut into chunks

1 medium onion, sliced

1 clove garlic, chopped

4 tomatoes, about 300g (9½oz), halved

1 sprig fresh rosemary

2 tablespoons olive oil

2 teaspoons cider vinegar

Preheat the oven to 200°C/400°F/Gas 6.

Season the fish with freshly ground black pepper and lemon juice, then cover the fish and leave to one side.

Put the vegetables and herbs in an ovenproof dish and toss them in the olive oil, vinegar and some more black pepper. Roast uncovered for 30 minutes, stirring a couple of times.

Brush the fish with olive oil and lay it on top of the vegetables. Cook in the oven for a further 5–10 minutes until the fish is just cooked. Serve immediately with a green leaf salad.

Mediterranean braised chicken

This recipe relies on good-quality ingredients for its delicious taste, so use the best olives available and pick ripe, juicy tomatoes. Keep any leftovers in the fridge and eat them cold for lunch the next day. Serves two.

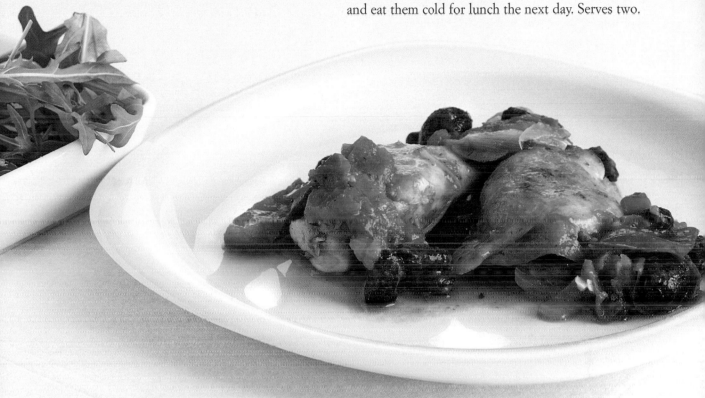

2 complete chicken legs (thigh and leg)

1 small onion, finely sliced

3 ripe medium tomatoes, sliced, or 400g (14oz) can tomatoes

1 teaspoon mixed "Herbes de Provence"

Juice of ½ lemon

60g (2oz) black olives

100g (4oz) cooked or canned red kidney beans

250ml (9fl oz) stock, either chicken or vegetable

Skin and joint the chicken legs. Lightly brown the chicken pieces in a tablespoon of olive oil over a high heat in a shallow casserole or a frying pan with a lid. Once browned, lift the chicken from the pan and put to one side.

Add a little more oil if necessary and gently soften the onion and tomato, together with the herbs and lemon juice, for five minutes. Add the olives and beans and 50ml (2fl oz) of the stock, then season with black pepper to taste.

Add the chicken joints, cover and cook over a very low heat for about 45 minutes until the chicken is cooked and tender. Top up with stock if necessary. The slow cooking will allow the chicken to fully absorb the flavours. Serve with a mixed leaf salad.

Oriental chicken

Allow at least half an hour between preparing the ingredients and cooking the chicken so that it can absorb the flavours of the marinade. Serves two.

1 small bunch fresh coriander leaves, roughly chopped

2 garlic cloves, roughly chopped

2 chillis, with or without seeds, roughly chopped

2.5cm (1in) ginger root, grated

Juice and zest of 1 lime

4 tablespoons light soy sauce

Freshly ground black pepper

2 chicken breasts, skinned and lightly scored

Place all the ingredients except the chicken breasts in a bowl, season with black pepper and mix well. Lay each chicken breast on a large piece of foil and rub the mixture over the chicken. Seal the foil, making two parcels, and leave to one side to marinate for at least 30 minutes.

Preheat the oven to 200°C/400°F/Gas 6.

Bake the chicken in the foil for 30 minutes, or until the meat is cooked. Transfer the chicken to two plates and serve with a green leaf salad.

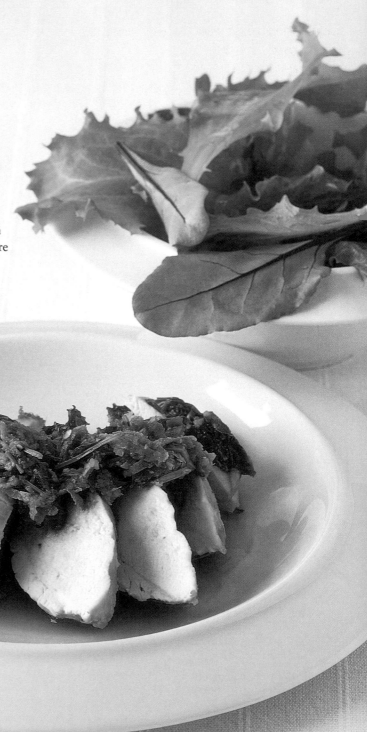

Lime chicken with a bean salad

The crisp, light flavours of a bean salad complement the citrus tang of this chicken recipe well. Serves two.

2 skinned chicken breasts, about 100g (4oz) for each portion

Juice and zest of 2 fresh limes

2 cloves garlic, finely chopped

1 handful oyster mushrooms, roughly chopped

1 handful fresh coriander leaves, roughly chopped

Cut the chicken breasts into strips about 1cm (⅓in) thick. Combine in a shallow bowl with the lime juice and zest, chopped garlic and a seasoning of freshly ground pepper. Leave to one side for about 15 minutes to allow the chicken to absorb the flavours.

Heat two tablespoons of olive oil in a wok or frying pan over a high heat. Remove the chicken from the marinade and stir-fry it in the hot oil. Reduce the heat, add the marinade and cook for five minutes. Add the mushrooms and coriander, cook for another minute or so and then serve with the bean salad.

Salad

100g (4oz) fine green beans, topped and tailed

100g (4oz) mangetout, shredded diagonally

100g (4oz) bean-sprouts

½ small red onion, finely sliced in rings

A handful of fresh coriander leaves, chopped

Steam the green beans and mangetout for three minutes or so. Then drain and run under cold water to refresh the vegetables. Tip them into a bowl, add the other ingredients and dress with an oriental salad dressing (see p.117).

Classic guacamole

Eat this creamy dip with various raw crudités such as mushrooms, carrots, spring onions, cherry tomatoes, red or yellow peppers and celery. Serves two.

2 ripe avocados

2 teaspoons grated onion

1 tablespoon mixed pumpkin, sunflower and sesame seeds

1 small clove garlic, crushed

2 teaspoons lemon juice

2 teaspoons olive oil

A pinch of cayenne pepper

A dash of Worcestershire sauce

A dash of Tabasco

Mash the avocados with the onion, seeds, garlic, lemon juice and olive oil in a small bowl. Add a seasoning of black pepper, cayenne pepper, Worcestershire sauce and Tabasco to taste.

Cover tightly with cling film and leave in the fridge for half an hour to let the flavours develop.

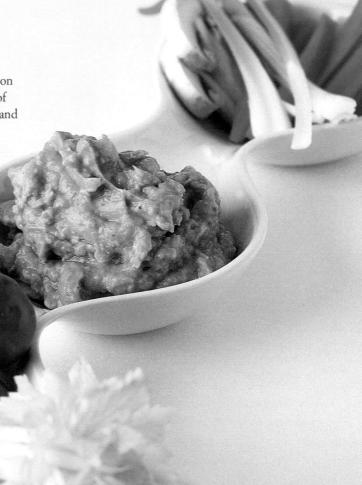

Fruit smoothie

Adapt this recipe to include seasonal fruits such as blackberries, peaches, fresh apricots and plums according to your preference. Keep any extra portions in the fridge for up to 24 hours. Serves two.

500g (16oz) live natural yoghurt

1 apple, peeled and cored

1 large ripe pear, peeled and cored

2 tablespoons pumpkin seeds

A good pinch of ground cinnamon

Put the yoghurt, apple, pear and pumpkin seeds into a food processor and blend until smooth. Pour into large mugs, top with cinnamon and serve.

Have a delicious **protein-rich** smoothie as a **refreshing** mid-morning or mid-afternoon **snack**

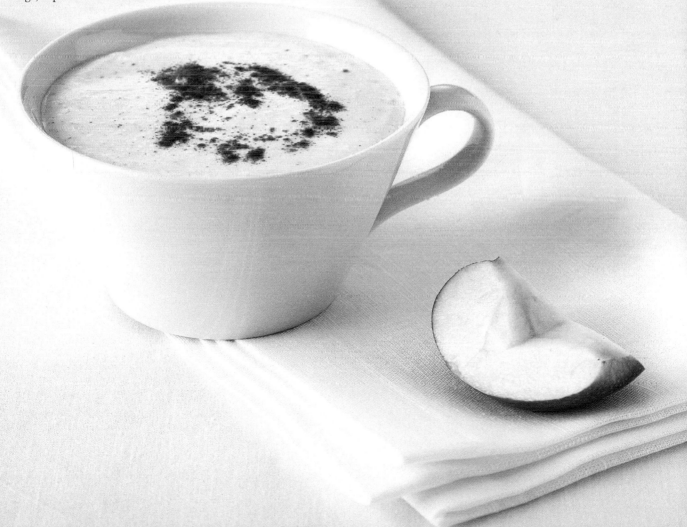

Hard-boiled eggs with crudités

Keep this snack in an airtight container in the fridge for up to two days. If you are a vegan, substitute the eggs with small chunks of firm tofu. Serves two.

6 quails' eggs or 2 hens' eggs

8 black olives

Approximately 250g (9oz) of a selection of raw vegetables – for example, carrots, broccoli, cauliflower, peppers, cherry tomatoes, cucumber, or celery – in small, almost bite-sized pieces

Hard-boil the eggs and allow to cool. Either leave the eggs whole in their shells, or remove the shells and cut the eggs into quarters. Arrange the eggs on a plate with the olives and raw vegetables and serve.

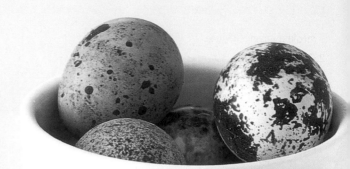

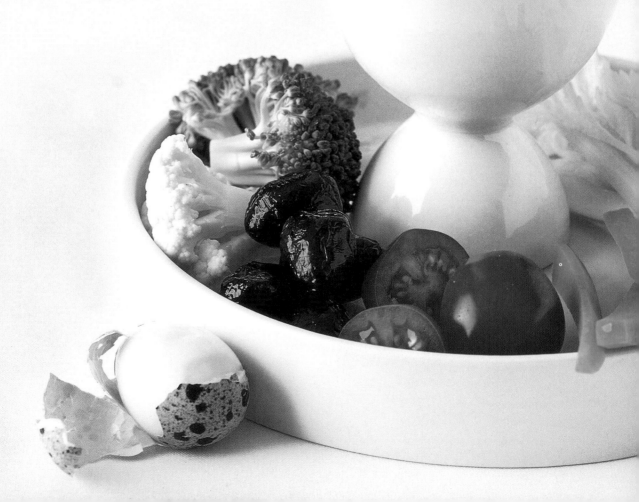

Vegetable omelette

Eat one serving of this omelette while hot, then keep the other portion in the fridge for up to two days to be eaten cold. Serves two.

1 medium onion, chopped

250g (9oz) spinach after removing any thick stems, rinsed and roughly torn if using mature spinach

2 medium tomatoes, peeled and chopped

A good grating of nutmeg

100g (4oz) canned chick-peas or flageolet beans

4 large eggs

A few stalks of watercress as a garnish

Soften the onion in a tablespoon of olive oil over a low heat in a large saucepan. Add the spinach, tomatoes and nutmeg and cook until most of the liquid has evaporated. Then add the chick-peas or beans.

Lightly whisk the eggs and season with freshly ground black pepper. Place a large frying pan over a low heat and add one tablespoon of olive oil. When the oil is hot, pour in half of the egg mixture, immediately followed by the vegetables and the rest of the eggs. Stir gently, cover with a lid and cook over a low heat for 10 minutes or so until set.

Brown the top under a medium grill. Turn out onto a plate, slice like a cake and serve with a garnish of watercress.

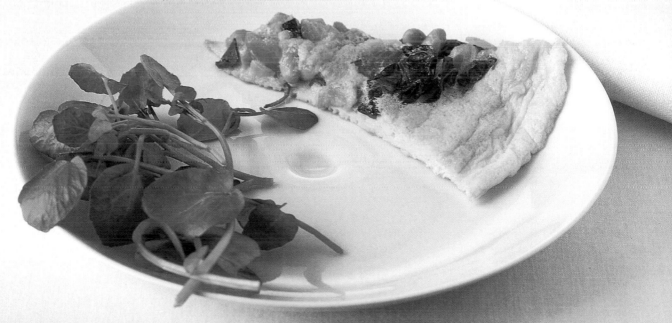

Glossary

Adrenaline

A hormone secreted by the adrenal glands (located above the kidneys) in response to low blood-glucose levels, exercise or stress. Adrenaline causes an increase in blood-sugar levels by breaking down glycogen stores to glucose in the liver, encouraging the release of fatty acids from body tissue, causing blood vessels to dilate and increasing cardiac output.

Amino acids

Amino acids form the basic constituents of proteins. There are nine essential amino acids that cannot be produced by the body and must be supplied by food, although the ninth is only considered essential for children.

Bacteria

Micro-organisms found in soil, air, water and food. Some bacteria are harmful and cause disease, others are beneficial, including many of those that live in the intestine and which help to break down food for digestion.

Blood-glucose levels

The concentration of glucose in the blood.

Cardiovascular

Relating to the heart and blood vessels.

Chyme

The pulpy, acidic, semi-liquid product of partly digested food that passes from the stomach to the small intestine.

Complex carbohydrate

A food containing insoluble fibre, which helps to slow down the process of digestion.

Diuretic effect

Increases the rate of urination, generally decreasing water retention.

Enzyme

A protein molecule that acts as a catalyst in bringing about biological reactions in the body. Enzymes are essential for normal function.

Essential fats

Fats that are essential to the normal functioning of the body, but which cannot be created by the body and so have to be derived from foods. Omega-3 essential fats are found in oily fish, such as mackerel, salmon, herring, tuna and sardines, and also in flax and hemp seeds. Omega-6 oils are found in most seeds and nuts except peanuts.

Fibre

Mostly derived from plant cell walls, fibre is not broken down by digestive enzymes but may be partly digested by beneficial bacteria in the gut. Fibre is essential for good digestive health: insoluble fibre provides bulk to the faeces and so helps to prevent constipation; soluble fibre helps to reduce blood-cholesterol levels and eliminate toxins and excess hormones.

Free radical

A naturally occurring, short-lived, highly unstable molecule that is usually produced when chemical reactions occur in the body. In its search for stability it will "steal" an electron from another molecule, causing it to become a free radical. This results in a cascade of free radical activity, which can result in the deterioration of tissue and degeneration associated with ageing, cancer, Alzheimer's, Parkinson's disease and arthritis, amongst many. Stress, pollution, poor diet, excessive sun exposure, smoking, radiation and illness all increase the build-up of free radicals.

Gliadin

A protein that constitutes gluten. Intolerance to gliadin is known as coeliac disease.

Glucose

A simple form of sugar, also known as a monosaccharide. It occurs naturally in various foods – for example, in some fruits – and is the body's main source of fuel. Carbohydrates are broken down into glucose by the body. However, body cells cannot use glucose without the help of insulin.

Gluten

An insoluble protein group that is found in wheat, rye, barley and oats. Gluten is the mixture of proteins, which includes gliadin, to which coeliacs are intolerant.

Glycaemic index

The glycaemic index ranks foods on a scale of 1–100 on how they affect blood-glucose levels. This index measures how much blood sugar increases in the two or three hours after eating. Foods that are broken down quickly during the process of digestion have the highest GI values (70 and above) – they make blood-glucose levels rise high quickly. Foods that are broken down slowly, releasing glucose gradually into the bloodstream, have low GI scores (under 55).

Hydrochloric acid

Hydrochloric acid, or stomach acid, is the acid component of gastric juice. It plays a number of important roles in the process of digestion, including creating the right acidic environment for protein digestion to occur and killing many pathogens present in food.

Insulin

The hormone insulin is produced by the pancreas and helps glucose to enter the body's cells where it is used up as fuel. Insulin is also a storage hormone in that it will cause any excess glucose that is not needed immediately for energy to be stored as glycogen in the liver or muscles, or converted to fat and stored in body tissue.

Irritable bowel syndrome (IBS)

Irritable bowel syndrome, also known as spastic colon, is a common disorder whereby the regular waves of muscular movement along the intestines become uncoordinated. This disruption, involving both the small intestine and the colon, results in a variety of symptoms in all areas of the digestive tract, including intermittent diarrhoea and constipation, cramp-like abdominal pain and swelling of the abdomen.

Metabolic rate

The energy required to keep the body functioning while at rest.

Metabolism

The "burning" of glucose in body cells to produce energy.

Minerals

Substances, such as calcium, magnesium and iron, that are naturally found in various foods and which are required by the body for the maintenance of good health. A balanced, healthy diet usually contains all the minerals the body requires.

Mitochondria

Found in the cytoplasm of every cell in the body. Due to their role in the production of energy-molecules, known as ATP, mitochondria are considered the "powerhouses" of cells.

Nutrients

Vital substances required by all living organisms for survival.

Organic produce

Food that has been produced using farming methods that severely restrict the use of artificial chemical fertilizers and pesticides, and animals reared without the routine use of drugs, antibiotics and wormers common in intensive livestock farming. Any organic product sold in the UK must, by law, display a certification symbol or number: the Soil Association's organic symbol is the UK's official certification mark.

Osteoporosis

A condition in which the density of bones declines, making them brittle and prone to fracture. The mineral calcium is essential for bone health.

Pathogen

Any micro-organism that causes disease, for example, a parasite.

Parasite

An organism that lives off and obtains food from another organism or host. Giardia is an example of a parasite that may be found in the gut.

Protein

A complex compound, made of carbon, hydrogen, oxygen and nitrogen and often sulphur, which is essential to all living things.

Protein is required for growth and repair and is broken down into amino acids by the body.

Saliva

An alkaline liquid secreted by the salivary glands into the mouth. Saliva lubricates food, helping in the process of chewing and swallowing, and contains an enzyme that helps to break down the starch in foods. It also has antibacterial properties.

Simple carbohydrate

A food that yields simple sugars, which are broken down rapidly into glucose by the body.

Saturated fats

Saturated fats are primarily animal fats that are solid at room temperature. Such fats are found in meat and dairy produce. Coconut oil is the only vegetable oil that contains a significant amount of saturated fats. Saturated fats have been shown to raise the levels of "bad" LDL (low-density lipoprotein) cholesterol in the blood.

Stimulants

Substances, including caffeine, found in foods and drinks, such as chocolate and fizzy drinks, that stimulate the production of adrenaline from the adrenal glands. Under normal circumstances, this release of adrenaline prepares the body for the "flight or fight" response syndrome, causing – among many things – the heart to beat faster. If adrenaline is overproduced because stimulant foods have been consumed, this may lead to fatigue and blood-glucose imbalances in the body.

Type 2 diabetes

Diabetes mellitus is a condition in which blood-glucose levels can become dangerously high because the body cannot utilize glucose properly. Excess blood-glucose levels (hyperglycaemia) can result in long-term damage to the eyes, kidneys, nerves, heart and major arteries. There are two principal types of diabetes: insulin-dependent Type 1 diabetes, and non-insulin dependent Type 2 diabetes, also known as adult-onset diabetes. In Type 2 diabetes the body cannot make

enough insulin, or cell receptors do not respond to insulin (also known as insulin resistance). This type of diabetes usually occurs in people over the age of 40, although it is becoming increasingly common in the younger population due to an increase in high-sugar, refined carbohydrate diets – even teenagers are now being diagnosed.

Villi

Fine, finger-like protrusions that cover the lining of the small intestines and which help to increase the surface area, thereby increasing the ability of the intestine to absorb nutrients.

Vitamins

Groups of complex organic substances, found in many different foods, that are essential in small amounts for the normal functioning of the body. There are 13 vitamins, and with the exception of vitamin D and niacin, which can be generated by the body, vitamins must be obtained from your diet. A varied diet will contain adequate amounts of all the vitamins.

Yeast

A single cell organism used in some food industry processes such as baking, brewing and winemaking. Some yeasts become pathogens once inside the body (for example, *Candida albicans*, which causes thrush) and may cause infection in any open canal in the body such as the vagina, ear, or mouth. Excess sugar, alcohol, stress, and antibiotics can cause a proliferation in pathogenic yeasts.

Useful addresses and websites

Please note that, due to the fast-changing nature of the worldwide web, some websites may be out of date by the time you read this.

ORGANIZATIONS IN THE UK AND THE REPUBLIC OF IRELAND

The British Allergy Foundation
Deepdene House
30 Belgrove Road
Welling, Kent DA16 3PY
Allergy helpline: 020 8303 8583
www.allergyfoundation.com

British College of Nutrition and Health
PO Box 43807
London NW6 3WQ
tel: 020 7372 5740
www.bcnh.co.uk

British Heart Foundation
14 Fitzhardinge Street
London W1H 6DH
www.bhf.org.uk

Coeliac Society of Ireland
Carmichael House
4 North Brunswick Street
Dublin 7
Ireland
tel: (01) 872 1471
www.coeliac@iol.ie

Coeliac UK
PO Box 220
High Wycombe
Bucks HP11 2HY
tel: 0870 444 8804
www.coeliac.co.uk
Charity supporting people with gluten intolerance.

Digestive Disorders Foundation
3 St Andrews Place
London NW1 4LB
tel: 020 7486 0341
www.digestivedisorders.org.uk

The Food Doctor
76–78 Holland Park Avenue
London W11 3RB
tel: 0800 093 5877
www.thefooddoctor.com

Heart UK
7 North Road
Maidenhead
Berkshire SL6 1PE
tel: 01628 628 638
www.heartuk.org.uk
Organization supporting and advising anyone wishing to reduce the risks of heart disease.

The IBS Network
Northern General Hospital
Sheffield S5 7AU
www.ibsnetwork.org.uk
For enquiries relating to gut reaction and IBS Network publications.

Institute of Optimum Nutrition
13 Blades Court
Deodar Road
Putney, London SW15 2NU
tel: 020 8877 9993
www.ion.ac.uk

Irish Diabetic Association
76 Lower Gardiner Street
Dublin 1
tel: (01) 836 3022
www.diabetes.ie

Irish Heart Foundation
4 Clyde Road. Ballsbridge
Dublin 4
tel: (01) 668 5001
www.irishheart.ie

Irish Nutrition and Dietetic Institute
Ashgrove House
Kill Avenue
Dun Laoghaire
Co. Dublin
info@indie.ie

National Association for Colitis and Crohn's Disease
4 Beaumont House
Sutton Road, St Albans
Herts AL1 5HH
tel: 0845 130 2233
www.nacc.org.uk

National Osteoporosis Society
Manor Farm
Skinner's Hill
Camerton, Bath BA2 OPJ
tel: 01761 471771
www.nos.org.uk

Organic Soil Association
Bristol House
40–56 Victoria Street
Bristol BS1 6BY
tel: 0117 929 0661
www.soilassociation.org
Campaigning and certification organization for organic food and farming.

www.gymguide.co.uk
Directory of health, fitness, sports and leisure clubs in the UK.

www.lactose.co.uk
Information on lactose intolerance, milk allergies and IBS.

ORGANIZATIONS IN AUSTRALIA

Allergy, Sensitivity and Environmental Health Association
PO Box 96
Margate QLD 4019
tel: 07 3284 8742
www.asehaqld.org.au

Australian Crohn's and Colitis Association
PO Box 497
13/96 Manchester Rd
Moroolbark VIC 3138
tel: 03 9726 9008
www.acca.net.au
Provides helpful information and links about colitis and Crohn's disease

Blackmores
23 Roseberry St
Balgowlah NSW 2093
Advisory service tel: 1800 803 760
www.blackmores.com.au
Website has online health experts and advice about numerous dietary problems and herbal supplements.

Coeliac Society of Australia
Unit 1/306 Victoria Ave Chatswood
NSW 2067
tel: 02 9411 4100
www.coeliac.org.au

Diabetes Australia
GPO Box 3156
Canberra ACT 2601
tel: 1300 136 588
www.diabetesaustralia.com.au

Gut Foundation
c/o Gastrointestinal Unit
The Prince of Wales Hospital
Randwick NSW 2031
tel: 02 9382 2789
www.gut.nsw.edu.au

Irritable Bowel Information and Support Association of Australia
PO Box 5044
Manly QLD 4179
tel: 07 3893 1131
www.ibis-australia.org.au

Nutrition Australia (Victoria)
c/o Caulfield General Medical Centre
260 Kooyong Rd
Caulfield VIC 3162
tel: 03 9528 2453
www.nutritionaustralia.org

www.foodwatch.com.au
Comprehensive website about nutrition and diet.

www.gastro.net.au
Authoritative resource in gastroenterology – online information service for patients and health professionals written by experienced gastroenterologists.

Index

Page numbers in *italics* indicate recipes.

About the author

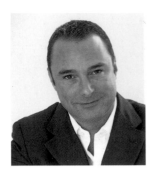

Ian Marber MBANT Dip ION
Nutrition consultant, author, broadcaster and health journalist

Ian studied at London's renowned Institute for Optimum Nutrition, and now heads The Food Doctor clinic at Notting Hill, London. He contributes regularly to many of Britain's leading magazines and newspapers, including *Marie Claire, Red, Attitude, The Daily Express, Evening Standard* and *ES*. In addition, he is an advisor and contributing editor for *Healthy* and *Here's Health*, two of Britain's most influential health magazines. Ian is also a sought-after guest on national television, appearing regularly on the BBC, Channel 4, ITN News and GMTV, as well as on many radio shows.

Undiagnosed food sensitivities in his twenties led to Ian becoming interested in nutrition. His condition was later identified as coeliac disease, a life-long intolerance to gluten. He is now an acknowledged expert on nutrition and digestion, and many of his clients are referred to The Food Doctor clinic by doctors and gastroenterologists.

Ian advises on all aspects of nutrition, and in particular on the impact that correct food choices can have. He is known by his clients to give highly motivational, positive advice that can make a real difference to their well-being.

His first book, *The Food Doctor – Healing Foods for Mind and Body,* was co-written with Vicki Edgson, in 1999. To date, it has sold around 300,000 copies and has been translated into nine languages. Ian's first solo title, *The Food Doctor in the City,* published in 2000, highlighted how to stay healthy in an urban environment. It was followed in 2001 by *In Bed with The Food Doctor*, which examines how nutrition can improve your libido and help you sleep well.

About The Food Doctor

Ian Marber and Vicki Edgson co-founded their Food Doctor nutrition practice in 1999 following the success of their original book, *The Food Doctor – Healing Foods for Mind and Body*. The consultancy is now a leading provider of nutritional information and services, including a busy clinic in West London and a network of nutrition consultants operating throughout the UK. The Food Doctor offers one-to-one consultations, workshops and lectures on a wide variety of subjects such as weight loss, children's nutrition, digestive health and stress management. It also works with major corporate clients to improve the health and well-being of their employees and frequently has to work with caterers to ensure a healthy choice of food is available.

The Food Doctor has developed its own food range to provide healthy meal solutions and snacks: all are designed to incorporate The Food Doctor ethos of balance and correct nutrition.

Acknowledgments

The author would like to thank:
Dame Shirley Bassey, Yvonne Bishop, Marylisa Browne, Simon Carey, Liz Claridge, Michael da Costa, Diane Filipovski, Stephen Garrett, Rebecca Haywood, Lisa Howells, Jani Isaacs, Shannon Leeman, Emma Lo, David Manning, Susie Perry, Rita Rakus, Stuart Scher, Antonia Smith, Robert Shrager, Mary Thomas, and, of course, my family.

Special thanks to Rowena Paxton for her delicious recipes, and to her family for being willing guinea pigs; to MC for her support and trust; and to the lovely Susannah Steel for her wonderful work in editing this book, and for making me laugh during stressful times.

The publisher would like to thank:
Penny Warren and Shannon Beatty for editorial assistance and Sarah Rock for design assistance.